T0292592

Surgery for Parkinson's Disease

Robert R. Goodman
Editor

Surgery for Parkinson's Disease

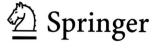 Springer

Editor
Robert R. Goodman
Hackensack Meridian School of Medicine
at Seton Hall University
Nutley, NJ
USA

ISBN 978-3-319-23692-6   ISBN 978-3-319-23693-3   (eBook)
https://doi.org/10.1007/978-3-319-23693-3

Library of Congress Control Number: 2018964422

This Springer imprint is published by the registered company Springer Nature Switzerland AG
The registered company address is: Gewerbestrasse 11, 6330 Cham, Switzerland

To Sarah, your lifelong love and support have been essential to all that I have accomplished.

Acknowledgment

I am extremely grateful to my colleagues, who have contributed to the chapters in this book. I greatly appreciate their hard work and patience, in sharing their knowledge and experience with those who share our interest, in offering surgery to benefit patients with disabling PD.

Introduction

The surgical treatment of Parkinson disease has been a focus of my neurosurgical practice since 1993. The practice has evolved significantly, over the past 25 years, transitioning from lesioning to deep brain stimulation therapy and with the development of various stereotactic techniques/options. For instance, my own practice has changed from using the traditional reusable stereotactic frame to a single-use custom-made 3D-printed plastic platform, to accurately guide electrodes to the chosen brain targets. I believe that my years of practice have taught me to appreciate the keys to the successful application of DBS therapy, for the treatment of patients with Parkinson disease. The most important of these is for the surgeon to be able to identify appropriate candidates for DBS therapy, specifically that means PD patients whose quality of life would be significantly improved, by the reduction of motor fluctuations or tremors. In addition, the surgeon must recognize that the single biggest morbidity of DBS implantation is the exacerbation of a preexisting cognitive decline/impairment. The second most important factor is for PD patients to have appropriate expectations for DBS therapy. Patients must understand that DBS therapy can improve management of dopa-responsive symptoms (e.g., motor fluctuations) and/or to reduce disabling hand tremors. It is equally important for patients to understand what DBS therapy is not expected to accomplish. That would include prevention of disease progression and improvement of non-dopa-responsive symptoms (e.g., on-freezing, deteriorating best on function, cognitive decline, and gait/balance dysfunction).

With the identification of appropriate DBS candidates and appropriate patient expectations, the key to successful DBS therapy depends on selecting the proper target and accomplishing accurate DBS lead implantation, without producing significant morbidity. In my own practice, I have favored the VIM thalamic target, for tremor-dominant patients and the STN target for patients disabled by motor fluctuations. I recommend the GPi target for a minority of patients, particularly those disabled by dopa-induced dyskinesias and or dystonias, who have not tolerated substantial escalation of dopa medication. I favor staged bilateral implantation for older patients and for patients with a concern for even mild or minor preoperative cognitive decline. I have found that the above can only be accomplished by a neurosurgeon working closely with movement disorder neurologists who have taken an interest in the surgical treatment of patients with PD.

Meticulous identification of the planned brain target is critical. This is dependent on obtaining proper imaging, which is facilitated by the elimination of patient movement during MR imaging. Over the past 7 years, I have obtained my preoperative MRIs with patients under general anesthesia. This guarantees excellent quality imaging. MRI is merged with a CT scan, to eliminate any concern about MRI distortion and to image the skull fiducial markers (used for the stereotactic platform). Proper targeting requires precise identification of the anterior and posterior commissures, correction of tilt, and adjustment based on individual patient anatomy. Trajectories are carefully planned, to avoid surface veins, or the traversing of sulci below the cortical surface or of the lateral ventricle. At surgery, I use a hair sparing prep. Patients greatly appreciate this, and it has not been associated with a significant infection rate. I have made two technical modifications to the implantation procedure, which I have found advantageous. I use a titanium plate to secure the lead to the skull (see Fig. 1). A groove is drilled into the outer table of the skull, adjacent to the burr hole, to allow this to be a very low-profile technique. I place a clip on the lead, while the lead is still held by the stereotactic apparatus, to allow me to confirm that the desired lead depth is maintained, until the lead is secured to the skull. A rectangular plate is used, to anchor the lead to the skull and to repair the burr hole defect. A silastic collar is placed over the lead, at the point of plate contact, to secure the lead. A second modification relates to the extension wire connection to the DBS lead. I drill a trough into the outer table of the skull (see Fig. 2a), to allow the extension to have a lower profile, and use a titanium mini-plate (see Fig. 2b), to secure the extension into the trough, to prevent migration into the soft tissues of the neck. I have found that patients appreciate both of these modifications.

Another important aspect of DBS therapy is to accurately identify the lead location, after implantation. I routinely obtain a post-implant thin-section head CT scan

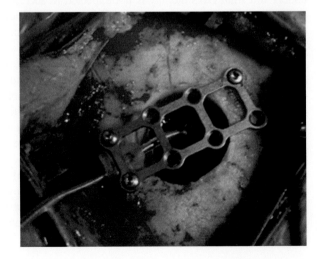

Fig. 1 The intraoperative photo depicts the titanium plate serving to anchor the DBS lead and to be a low-profile repair of the bur hole defect. Also seen are the clip on the lead (to maintain desired depth) and the silastic collar on the lead (to protect the lead from the titanium plate)

Fig. 2 Intraoperative photos demonstrate the trough drilled in the skull (to lower the profile of the connector) and the use of a titanium plate to secure the connector in the trough

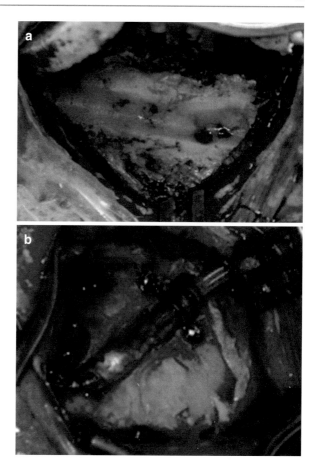

and merge it with the planning MRI, to confirm the location of the lead, relative to the planned target. This can also be accomplished with a postoperative brain MRI. In general, the lead must be within 2 mm of the planned target, to achieve the desired clinical benefit. If it is not within this margin, and clinical benefit is suboptimal, revision must be considered. Also, with my lead anchoring technique, if the depth is not as desired, the anchoring plate can be loosened and the depth easily adjusted, at the surgery for extension wire and IPG implantation.

It is important for DBS surgeons to monitor their results and to confirm that they are similar to results in the literature. In my own case, our group analyzed and reported the results of my first 100 STN DBS-implanted patients [1]. This is a very useful exercise, since it could identify issues that should be addressed.

Finally, one of my main reasons for creating this book is that I am convinced that surgical treatment, when performed properly, is extremely beneficial to appropriate patients with PD. Although surgical therapy has grown significantly over the last 20 years, I believe that it is an underutilized intervention, and I hope that its application will expand greatly, in the coming years. I am hopeful that this book will achieve its goal, to be a practical guide for neurosurgeons pursuing DBS therapy, and other modalities, for the treatment of patients with PD.

Reference

1. Goodman RR, Kim B, McClelland S III, Senatus PB, Winfield LM, Pullman SL, Yu Q, Ford B, McKhann GM II. Operative techniques and morbidity with sub-thalamic nucleus deep brain stimulation in 100 consecutive patients with advanced Parkinson Disease. J Neurol Neurosurg Psychiatry. 2006;77(1):12–7.

Contents

Contributors

Punit Agrawal Department of Neurology and Center for Neuromodulation, The Ohio State University Wexner Medical Center, Columbus, OH, USA

Ellen L. Air Department of Neurosurgery, Henry Ford Hospital, Detroit, MI, USA

G. H. Baltuch Department of Neurosurgery, University of Pennsylvania, Philadelphia, PA, USA

H. Bergman Department of Medical Neurobiology (Physiology), Institute of Medical Research Israel-Canada (IMRIC), Edmond and Lily Safra Center (ELSC) for Brain Research, The Hebrew University, Jerusalem, Israel

Department of Neurosurgery, Hadassah University Hospital, Jerusalem, Israel

Andrea Brock Department of Neurosurgery, University of Utah, Salt Lake City, UT, USA

R. Eitan Department of Medical Neurobiology (Physiology), Institute of Medical Research Israel-Canada (IMRIC), Edmond and Lily Safra Center (ELSC) for Brain Research, The Hebrew University, Jerusalem, Israel

Eric Hudgins Department of Neurosurgery, University of Pennsylvania, Philadelphia, PA, USA

Hubert H. Fernandez Cleveland Clinic, Neurologic Institute, Center for Neurological Restoration, Cleveland, OH, USA

Department of Neurology, Cleveland Clinic, Neurologic Institute, Cleveland, OH, USA

Kelly D. Foote University of Florida, Department of Neurosurgery, Gainesville, FL, USA

Carter S. Gerard Department of Neurosurgery, Swedish Neuroscience Institute, Seattle, WA, USA

Michal Gostkowski Cleveland Clinic, Neurologic Institute, Center for Neurological Restoration, Cleveland, OH, USA

Department of Neurology, Cleveland Clinic, Neurologic Institute, Cleveland, OH, USA

Fiona Gupta Department of Neurology, The Mount Sinai Hospital, New York, NY, USA

Ryder Gwinn Department of Neurosurgery, Swedish Neuroscience Institute, Seattle, WA, USA

Sameah Haider Department of Neurosurgery, Albany Medical Center, Albany, NY, USA

Melissa Hardy Department of Biology, Salt Lake Community College, Salt Lake City, UT, USA

Justin D. Hilliard University of Florida, Department of Neurosurgery, Gainesville, FL, USA

Paul House Department of Neurosurgery, University of Utah, Salt Lake City, UT, USA

Z. Israel Department of Neurosurgery, Hadassah University Hospital, Jerusalem, Israel

Vignessh Kumar Department of Neurosurgery, Albany Medical Center, Albany, NY, USA

Wendell Lake University of Wisconsin-Madison, Department of Neurosurgery, Madison, WI, USA

Steven Lange Department of Neurosurgery, Albany Medical Center, Albany, NY, USA

Andre G. Machado Department of Neurosurgery, Cleveland Clinic, Neurologic Institute, Cleveland, OH, USA

Cleveland Clinic, Neurologic Institute, Center for Neurological Restoration, Cleveland, OH, USA

Andres L. Maldonado-Naranjo Department of Neurosurgery, Cleveland Clinic, Neurologic Institute, Cleveland, OH, USA

Charles B. Mikell III Department of Neurosurgery, Stony Brook University Hospital, Stony Brook, NY, USA

Sean J. Nagel Department of Neurosurgery, Cleveland Clinic, Neurologic Institute, Cleveland, OH, USA

Cleveland Clinic, Neurologic Institute, Center for Neurological Restoration, Cleveland, OH, USA

Joseph S. Neimat Department of Neurological Surgery, University of Louisville, Louisville, KY, USA

Julie G. Pilitsis Department of Neurosurgery, Albany Medical Center, Albany, NY, USA

Department of Neuroscience and Experimental Therapeutics, Albany Medical Center, Albany, NY, USA

A. G. Ramayya Department of Neurosurgery, University of Pennsylvania, Philadelphia, PA, USA

Adolfo Ramirez-Zamora Department of Neurology, University of Florida, Gainesville, FL, USA

Richard Rammo Department of Neurosurgery, Henry Ford Hospital, Detroit, MI, USA

Jason M. Schwalb Department of Neurosurgery, Henry Ford West Bloomfield Hospital, West Bloomfield, MI, USA

Vishad Sukul Department of Neurosurgery, Albany Medical College, Albany, NY, USA

David Shin University of Florida, Department of Neurosurgery, Gainesville, FL, USA

Part I

The Current Practice of Surgery for PD

Indications for Deep Brain Stimulation Therapy in Parkinson's Disease

Andrea Brock, Melissa Hardy, and Paul House

Summary for the Clinician
- Progressive idiopathic Parkinson's disease is a movement disorder resulting from the death of dopamine-producing neurons in the substantia nigra.
- Diagnosis of PD requires bradykinesia and one of the following: Rigidity, rest tremor, or idiopathic postural instability.
- A single causative agent has not been identified. Most cases are idiopathic.
- The disease is invariably progressive. Motor symptoms progress from unilateral to bilateral, and nomotor symptoms generally develop following motor symptoms.

Background

Parkinson's disease (PD) affects approximately 0.3% of the general population and 1% of people over 60 years old with an incidence of 8–18 per 100,000 person years [1, 2]. As life expectancy increases, the number of people with PD is projected to double by 2030 [3]. The onset of PD is rare before age 50 with the incidence becoming higher with age.

A. Brock · P. House (✉)
Department of Neurosurgery, University of Utah, Salt Lake City, UT, USA
e-mail: paul.house@hsc.utah.edu

M. Hardy
Department of Biology, Salt Lake Community College, Salt Lake City, UT, USA

© Springer Nature Switzerland AG 2019
R. R. Goodman (ed.), *Surgery for Parkinson's Disease*,
https://doi.org/10.1007/978-3-319-23693-3_1

Symptoms and Diagnosis

There is no definitive test for the diagnosis of PD. Because a variety of diseases can create Parkinsonian features not caused by idiopathic PD, several diagnostic criteria have been proposed. The Parkinson's Disease Society of the UK established widely cited clinical criteria to create a pathological brain bank. Symptoms must include bradykinesia in addition to rigidity, rest tremor, or idiopathic postural instability. A history of repeated strokes, head injury, sustained remission, or lack of dopamine response excludes the diagnosis. Supportive criteria such as unilateral onset, excellent dopamine response, and a long clinical course can allow for a definite diagnosis [4]. Nonmotor symptoms, such as autonomic insufficiency, sleep disorders, and cognitive difficulties, typically develop after the appearance of motor symptoms.

The majority of patients with clinically diagnosed PD do not have a family history of PD. An estimated 5–10% of cases have a monogenic cause [5]. Recent studies have identified several alleles that confer a risk of PD. These, combined with environmental insult, probably contribute to a large number of idiopathic PD cases [6]. The variation in symptoms and progression of PD suggests that it is a heterogeneous disease, which highlights the need for careful diagnosis and follow-up before undertaking surgical therapy [7, 8].

Disease Progression

PD is a progressive disorder. A diagnosis of typical idiopathic PD connotes a continual, although nonlinear, progression of both motor and nonmotor symptoms. Symptoms are typically unilateral at first and become bilateral as the disease progresses. The Unified Parkinson's Disease Rating Scale (UPDRS) is the most widely used scale to track the severity and progression of PD symptoms [9]. The total scale (score range 0–199) incorporates scores for activities of daily living and mood, as well as movement scores. Using the total UPDRS to track the progression of PD, Jankovic reported a worsening of scores by 1.58 points per year when patients were not taking medication [10]. Using this total UPDRS score, a minimal clinically important change in early PD is calculated to be 3.5 points [11].

PD confers an increased risk of mortality. In an extensive meta-analysis covering studies performed after the introduction of levodopa therapy, patients with PD were shown to have a mortality rate 1.5 times that of the general population. This risk increases over time, with a 5% decrease in survival for every year after diagnosis [12]. Life expectancy after diagnosis ranges from 6.9 to 14.3 years.

Pathophysiology

The pathophysiology underlying the movement disorder associated with PD is degeneration of dopamine-producing neurons within the substantia nigra pars compacta. These neurons degenerate with age more extensively in PD patients than in the general population. According to the classical "rate model" of basal ganglia function, dopamine acts to allow stimulation of the cerebral cortex by thalamocortical neurons, allowing normal movement. Dopamine from the substantia nigra is delivered to the striatum, where it acts through two pathways. The direct pathway facilitates the movement by relieving inhibition of thalamocortical neurons from the internal segment of the globus pallidus (GPi). The indirect pathway inhibits movement by activating neurons of the subthalamic nucleus (STN) that activate the inhibitory neurons of the GPi. When dopamine is present, the direct pathway is stimulated, while the indirect pathway is inhibited. In PD, dopamine is depleted, which reduces activity of the direct pathway and boosts the inhibitory effect of the indirect pathway [13].

The rate model from which these pathways are derived, while necessarily simplified, has been used for the study and treatment of PD. Carlsson first demonstrated the efficacy of levodopa in restoring motor function to animals treated with reserpine, a drug that depletes brain dopamine and causes Parkinsonism, in 1957. These findings were extended to human patients over the next decade [14].

Multiple potential causes for idiopathic PD have been proposed, and a single causative agent has not been identified; however, a pathological accumulation of the α-synuclein protein in the form of Lewy bodies is diagnostic of the disease, and it has been proposed that the α-synuclein might behave in a prion-like manner [15]. Braak et al. proposed a unifying pathological staging system for PD based on the location and extent of Lewy body involvement [16]. Early PD is characterized by involvement of the lower brainstem and olfactory area, while later stages show involvement of the substantia nigra pars compacta and eventually the hippocampus and higher neocortical structures. While the exact histological progression has been debated, and likely varies based on clinic subtypes, the disease is predictably progressive [17].

Summary for the Clinician
- Levodopa therapy greatly improves motor symptoms. However, it is usually associated with the development of dyskinesia and fluctuations in therapeutic benefit over time.
- Careful medication adjustments and the use of medical adjuvants are often sufficient to minimize motor fluctuations for years after diagnosis.
- Deep brain stimulation therapy of the GPi or STN can dramatically improve motor fluctuations and minimize "off" time.

Medical Therapy

Since its introduction in the late 1960s, levodopa has been the most symptomatically efficacious oral medication to treat PD-related motor symptoms. Levodopa therapy is commonly prescribed in a dual formulation with a peripheral L-aromatic amino acid decarboxylase (L-AAAD) inhibitor such as carbidopa to prevent the peripheral breakdown of levodopa [18, 19]. This combination increases the availability of levodopa to cross through the blood–brain barrier where it is converted into dopamine. This increase in striatal dopamine results in the improvement of motor symptoms [20].

Most patients treated with levodopa for 5–10 years develop motor complications, especially dyskinesia. There are both clinical and experimental animal model data suggesting dyskinesia may be a side effect of levodopa therapy [21–23]. On the other hand, the development of dyskinesia may simply represent a stage of disease progression that will occur regardless of timing of dopamine therapy. Ahlskog and Muenter [24] found that about 40% of patients develop motor fluctuations and about 40% develop dyskinesias within 4–6 years after beginning levodopa therapy. They also found that, among patients who developed PD before the availability of levodopa, 50% of patients developed dyskinesias within 5–6 months of beginning therapy, suggesting the duration of PD itself might be the critical factor in dyskinesia development. Cilia et al. recently reported similar findings. These researchers compared a group of patients in Ghana with a group of Italian patients in a cross-sectional case-controlled manner. The Ghanaian patients, on average, had much longer disease duration prior to the initiation of levodopa therapy (4.9 versus 1.6 years), and the group of levodopa-naïve patients developed dyskinesia only 6 months after initiation of therapy [25]. These studies suggest that dyskinesia is a common symptom in later-stage PD.

The use of high-dose levodopa early after the diagnosis of PD may particularly correlate with the earlier development of motor fluctuations and dyskinesia. Because of this concern, many neurologists delay initiation of dopamine replacement therapy (DRT). Pramipexole and ropinirole (dopamine agonists) have shown good efficacy as initial monotherapy alternatives to DRT. Regardless of timing of initiation, however, PD patients will eventually require and greatly benefit from DRT. Most will later develop motor fluctuations, and dopamine agonists are also effective at reducing "off" time [26–28]. Entacapone (a catechol-O-methyl transferase inhibitor) and rasagiline (a monoamine oxidase inhibitor) have also both been clearly shown to reduce "off" time. Cabergoline and selegiline have also shown some efficacy for this indication [28].

The careful adjustment and use of oral medications are often sufficient to minimize motor fluctuations and dyskinesias for some time. The use of continuously delivered carbidopa–levodopa directly into the jejunum is another recent development in medical therapy. Direct continuous delivery has been shown to improve "off" time by about 2 h per day and decrease "on" time accompanied by dyskinesias by approximately 2 h per day [29]. This form of therapy, however, requires the maintenance of a percutaneous jejunostomy access tube and continuous wearing of an infusion pump, limiting its application for younger and more physically active patients.

Despite expert management and the use of complex medication dosing schedules, fluctuations in motor symptoms can become disabling. At this point, deep brain stimulation should be considered to control these symptoms and to minimize "off" time.

Surgical Therapy

Although DBS has been widely clinically available as therapy for less than 20 years, two of the targets used for stimulation were discovered decades ago and extensively used in lesioning procedures. As reviewed by Guridi and Lozano, the identification of the modern pallidotomy target was based on both anatomical considerations and surgical discoveries [30]. Thalamotomy and pallidotomy were extensively used to improve motor symptoms, primarily tremor, prior to the development of levodopa therapy [31].

The development of the third widely used target, the subthalamic nucleus (STN), is more recent. The Lasker-DeBakey Clinical Medical Research Award was presented in 2014 to Benabid and DeLong for the development of STN DBS. Benabid, a neurosurgeon, observed that high-frequency (>100 Hz) stimulation of the ventral intermediate nucleus (VIM) thalamus reduced tremors. (Stimulation was performed as prelesioning testing during thalamotomy procedures.) DeLong, a neurologist, extensively investigated firing patterns of neurons in the basal ganglia and described the concept of parallel cognitive and motor systems [32]. He described excessive and abnormally patterned firing of a basal ganglia output nucleus (the STN) and later showed that lesioning of the STN could dramatically improve tremor, rigidity, and bradykinesia in an MPTP (1-methyl-4-phenyl-1,2,3,6-tetrahydropyridine) nonhuman primate model of PD [33]. Building on DeLong's mechanistic insights into PD, Benabid implanted the first DBS system into the STN in a human [34]. After the dramatic success of high-frequency stimulation, the US Food and Drug Administration approved the therapy in 2002.

Mechanism of Action of DBS

How DBS alleviates Parkinsonian symptoms is not entirely understood. DBS produces a clinical effect similar to that obtained by lesioning a target structure, suggesting an overall inhibitory effect on neuronal activity. Conflicting evidence, however, suggests DBS can drive local neuronal firing [35].

A large body of work evaluating STN DBS has focused on abnormally synchronous neuronal activity. Both the STN and primary motor cortex in humans have β oscillations (13–30 Hz), which are thought to be related to bradykinesia because they are suppressed by movement, dopaminergic medications, and DBS [36, 37]. On the basis of unique human simultaneous basal ganglia and motor cortex recordings, Shimamoto et al. [38] proposed that the clinical hypokinesia seen in PD is the result of increased β synchrony in the motor cortex secondary to pathological β oscillations sent from the STN.

There is evidence that DBS causes activation of efferent and afferent axons as well as axons passing near the locations of lead placement while also producing a "lesion-like" effect. Integrating these conflicting findings with the results of their own nonhuman primate investigations, Chiken and Nambu [39] proposed a common mechanism, whereby DBS inhibits information flow through the basal ganglia by interrupting coordinated input and output signals.

Goals of DBS

The benefits of DBS have been well established by large prospective and retrospective trials. For appropriately selected patients, DBS can provide profound improvement in the cardinal symptoms of PD—bradykinesia, tremor, and rigidity. DBS can also dramatically improve dyskinesia associated with dopamine therapy. DBS therapy has been shown to correlate with significant improvements in quality-of-life measures when prospectively compared with best medical therapy [40–45].

> **Summary for the Clinician**
> - DBS therapy has been extensively studied in large prospective and retrospective trials.
> - DBS dramatically reduces fluctuations in motor symptoms.
> - DBS provides profound reduction in tremor, bradykinesia, and medication-induced dyskinesia.
> - DBS has been shown to significantly improve quality of life when compared to continued best medical therapy without DBS.

Reduction in Motor Symptom Fluctuations

The primary goal of DBS therapy is an overall reduction in disability due to rapid fluctuations in an individual's ability to move well. Disability can be caused by relative undertreatment of symptoms, such as the re-emergence of bradykinesia as effective medication levels decline. Disability can also be caused by medication side effects, especially dyskinesia. A review of primarily retrospective studies noted an average reduction of 68% in "off" time [45] with DBS therapy. In a landmark prospective, randomized trial of STN DBS versus continued best medical therapy without DBS, Deuschl et al. [40] showed that patients obtained an additional 4.4 h of mobility not limited by dyskinesia and reduced periods of immobility by 4.2 h per day at the 6-month time point. This successful reduction in "off" symptoms has now been replicated in other prospective trials [41, 42, 46]. This is a significant effect, since a reduction of even 1.0 h of "off" time per day indicates a clinically important change [11].

Reduction in Tremor

Stimulation of the STN, GPi, or VIM thalamus can produce profound improvement in tremor. An open-label trial of thalamic stimulation in 73 patients with PD showed an improvement in contralateral tremor of >50% in 85% of individuals [47]. A systematic literature review of bilateral STN stimulation in 471 patients revealed an

81% reduction in tremor [44]. A prospective trial of STN stimulation similarly revealed a 75% tremor reduction in the medication "off" state [43]. Importantly, the reduction in tremor is seen independent of medication effect.

Reduction in Bradykinesia

Bradykinesia, or akinesia, is reduced with stimulation of the STN or GPi. The degree of bradykinesia reduction is in proportion to the reduction seen with the use of levodopa. A review of primarily retrospective studies found that a group of patients, who had an average of 57% preoperative reduction in bradykinesia in response to levodopa, showed a 46% improvement in bradykinesia during the medication "off" state in response to DBS at 6 months, 52% at 12 months, and 49% at 24 months [45]. Bradykinesia in the medication "on" state is not significantly improved and bradykinesia worsens over time with disease progression. For example, 8 years after DBS surgery, bradykinesia measured with UPDRS scale during the "on" medication and "on" DBS state (i.e., best possible function) had worsened from 7.4 to 14.7 [48].

Reduction of Dyskinesia

Patients with dyskinesia show marked improvement with DBS. In a review of 37 cohorts including 921 patients treated with bilateral STN DBS, Kleiner-Fisman et al. [45] found a reported 69% average reduction in dyskinesia. Reporting of dyskinesia was heterogeneous across studies, however, as UPDRS scores, the Abnormal Involuntary Movement Scale, the Dyskinesia Rating Scale, and patient diaries were variously used in the studies. In general, the reduction in dyskinesia seen with GPi stimulation is thought to be produced by a direct antidyskinetic effect, whereas the reduction in dyskinesia seen with STN stimulation is related to an overall reduction in dopaminergic medications.

Improvement in Quality of Life

Many studies evaluating the effectiveness of DBS have focused on the UPDRS-III subscales (range 0 to 108). These scales focus directly on movement symptoms, an area where the effects of DBS are clearly, and often quickly, evident. Patients, however, are primarily concerned about the overall effect of a therapy on their daily quality of life. After 6 months of therapy, Deuschl et al. [40] reported that quality of life (as measured with the Parkinson Disease Questionnaire (PDQ-39)) was improved by ~25% for patients treated with bilateral STN DBS. The VA cooperative trial reported improvements in most quality-of-life measures at 6-, 24-, and 36-month time points compared with baseline using either the STN or GPi as stimulation target [41]. Improvements in quality of life declined over time in these prospective studies, likely because quality-of-life measures are affected by both motor and nonmotor symptoms that inevitably progress.

> **Summary for the Clinician**
> - DBS does not reduce nonmotor symptoms such as cognition, depression, or autonomic instability.
> - Nonmotor symptoms are often severely disabling for patients.
> - While DBS improves quality of life, it does not slow the overall progression of Parkinson's disease.

Limitations of DBS

Whereas motor symptoms are usually greatly improved by DBS therapy, the nonmotor symptoms of PD and disease progression are generally not improved. Unfortunately, these nonmotor symptoms (such as cognitive decline, dysarthria, dysphasia, depression, mood lability, and autonomic instability) often produce severe disability, causing patients to seek DBS implantation. Appropriate counseling is needed for patients with these symptoms.

DBS Does Not Reduce Nonmotor Symptoms

It is generally agreed that nonmotor symptoms of PD are not improved with DBS and are not an appropriate indication for DBS therapy. While there have been concerns that DBS can worsen preexisting depression, several long-term trials have not revealed significant changes in depressive symptoms [43, 48, 49]. Likewise, despite concern that STN DBS might lead to an increased incidence of suicide, this was not seen in a prospective, randomized trial [50]. Nonmotor symptoms are sometimes attributable to medical therapy. For example, dopaminergic medications, especially dopamine agonists, can cause impulsive and compulsive behaviors such as compulsive buying, gambling, eating, and inappropriate sexual behavior [51]. DBS can be particularly useful to allow for medication reduction in these situations.

DBS Does Not Slow Progression of the Disease

Although most patients continue to experience benefit from DBS therapy for many years, there is no evidence that DBS slows the progression of PD. To date, long-term reports have focused on relatively early-onset PD patients. Even in these patients, who would be expected to have slower disease progression than average PD patients, motor and nonmotor symptoms worsen. Although patients treated with thalamic stimulation are able to maintain stable UPDRS-II scores, they require higher doses of levodopa 5 years after DBS placement [52]. Bang Henriksen et al. followed a group of patients 10 years after starting STN DBS therapy and found a steady progression of disease—including the development of dementia in 53% just over 5 years after surgery. Notably, these patients had an average disease duration of 25 years at the time of this follow-up [53].

Indications and Patient Selection

Patient selection is of the utmost importance when considering DBS therapy. An estimated 30% of DBS failures result from inappropriate surgical indications [54]. Patients who have a well-established PD diagnosis, who respond well to levodopa, and who have sufficiently disabling symptoms and/or drug side effects may be considered for surgery.

The patient selection process is best performed in a group model because many inclusion and exclusion criteria have both subjective and objective components. In general, the selection process should include evaluation by a movement disorders neurologist, a neurosurgeon, and a neuropsychologist or psychiatrist. Some centers include evaluation by a physical therapist. Given the degree of social limitations imposed by PD, the assistance of a patient coordinator and social worker support can also be invaluable.

The criteria established by the Centers for Medicare and Medicaid services for approval of DBS (Table 1.1) have been widely adopted by other insurance providers. At a practical level, these criteria serve as a reasonable benchmark for patient selection.

Table 1.1 Centers for Medicare and Medicaid services criteria for DBS for PD

Inclusion criteria	Exclusion criteria
Diagnosis of PD based on the presence of at least two cardinal PD features (tremor, rigidity, or bradykinesia)	Nonidiopathic PD or "Parkinson's plus" syndromes
Advanced idiopathic PD as determined by the use of Hoehn and Yahr stage or Unified Parkinson's Disease Rating Scale (UPDRS) part III motor subscale	Cognitive impairment, dementia, or depression that would be worsened by or would interfere with the patient's ability to benefit from DBS
L-dopa responsive with clearly defined "on" periods	Current psychosis, alcohol abuse, or other drug abuse
Persistent disabling PD symptoms or drug side effects (e.g., dyskinesias, motor fluctuations, or disabling "off" periods) despite optimal medical therapy	Structural lesions such as basal ganglionic stroke, tumor, or vascular malformation as etiology of the movement disorder
Willingness and ability to cooperate during conscious operative procedure, as well as during postsurgical evaluations, adjustments of medications and stimulator settings	Previous movement disorder surgery within the affected basal ganglion
	Significant medical, surgical, neurologic, or orthopedic comorbidities contraindicating DBS surgery or stimulation

Diagnosis of PD

Although PD is one of the most common neurodegenerative disorders, definite diagnosis still presents challenges. PD is a heterogeneous disease, and not all patients will have all symptoms, especially early in the course of the disease. Moreover, motor symptoms of PD are also features of other "Parkinson's Plus" syndromes, such as progressive supranuclear palsy, multiple systems atrophy, and dementia with Lewy bodies [55]. Unfortunately, even expert neurologists using the UK Parkinson's Disease Society Brain Bank Criteria for diagnosis were shown to only be accurate 82% of the time when the clinical diagnosis was later histologically evaluated by autopsy [56].

Surgery generally should not be considered for at least 5 years after the diagnosis of PD. The features that distinguish several of the "Parkinson's Plus" syndromes (such as early and severe balance difficulties, rapid cognitive worsening, and eye movement limitations) often present during this 5-year window, eliminating the diagnosis of idiopathic PD.

The Controlled Trial of Deep Brain Stimulation in Early Patients with Parkinson's Disease (EARLYSTIM) recently compared STN DBS treatment with best medical therapy and showed that DBS provided marked improvement in quality of life, motor disability, and activities of daily living [57]. The superiority of DBS therapy in this trial was pronounced and has led to concern that DBS will be suggested inappropriately for PD patients in an early stage of disease or who later are clearly shown not to suffer from PD [58]. Patients selected for the EARLYSTIM trial had been diagnosed with motor fluctuations for less than 3 years prior to enrollment and only needed to have carried a PD diagnosis for 4 years. Importantly, however, patients needed to show profound dopamine responsiveness (>50% improvement) and at the time of enrollment patients turned out to have carried a PD diagnosis for an average of 7.5 years. Patients were enrolled at Hoehn and Yahr stage 3 or less at the best "on" condition. (The Hoehn and Yahr scale was published in 1967 to codify disease progression and ranges from 1 to 5 [59].) The patients actually enrolled in the trial do not reflect those seen "early" after a diagnosis of PD so much as they reflect a well-chosen group who should, and did, respond well to DBS therapy. The study, and concerns raised by its title, help emphasize the need for a comprehensive team, including an expert movement disorders neurologist, to complete the DBS evaluation. Inappropriately offering surgery to patients only a few years after diagnosis essentially ensures that some patients without PD will be implanted, placing them operative risk with little potential benefit.

Disability

Patients with PD become candidates for surgery when motor fluctuations, dyskinesia, or dopamine-responsive symptoms become disabling. If dopamine-responsive symptoms are well controlled during the majority of the day, then DBS is not generally appropriate. Using the Hoehn and Yahr staging system, "advanced" PD is defined as stage 4 or 5 in the "off" medication state. (The scale was developed prior to the availability of DRT.). "Advanced" disease has not been defined specifically using the UPDRS-III scale (range 0–108), but operationally an "off" score of ≥30 is generally required to consider DBS implantation. As another reference point for consideration of DBS therapy, the VA Cooperative Study trial required patients to be Hoehn and Yahr ≥ stage 2 with persistent and disabling motor fluctuations and/or dyskinesia. More than 3 h per day of disability due to poor motor function was required for enrollment [41].

Levodopa Responsiveness

The response of disabling motor symptoms to levodopa is the strongest predictor of symptomatic response to DBS. Therefore, many centers use a levodopa challenge to grade levodopa responsiveness that includes assessing a patient who has not been taking medication for at least 12 h using the UPDRS-III score and then assessing again approximately 1 h after medication administration [60]. An improvement of at least 30% in UPDRS-III score is indicative of a predictably positive response to DBS [45]. Hourly patient diaries can also be helpful to establish the presence of clear "on" medication times when movement benefit is consistently noted.

Tremor is often unresponsive to levodopa administration. In patients who otherwise meet diagnostic criteria for PD and show good dopamine response to other cardinal features, a lack of tremor improvement does not preclude DBS therapy. In fact, tremor proves to be well treated with DBS regardless of preoperative "on/off" medication testing change [44, 47]. Dyskinesia is generally induced with levodopa therapy and likewise will be induced with "on/off" testing. The induction of dyskinesia can be seen as a secondary indication for DBS therapy.

Contraindications and Additional Considerations

Cognitive Impairment

Cognitive impairment is an intrinsic part of PD and likely develops as pathological Lewy body inclusions spread to involve memory circuitry such as the hippocampi [16]. DBS surgery and DBS therapy do not produce a cognitive improvement or decline in most patients, although STN DBS can be associated with verbal fluency impairment [61, 62]. There are not absolute established criteria for an acceptable level of preoperative cognitive dysfunction [63].

The Mattis Dementia Rating Scale (MDRS) is commonly used to screen for dementia (range 0–144). It has been shown that a cut-off score ≤ 123 reliably diagnoses dementia in PD patients [64]. A cut-off score ≥ 130 is commonly required of DBS candidates. Witt et al. [65] reviewed patients enrolled in a prospective STN DBS trial to evaluate how outcomes related to MDRS score. Patients were divided into quartiles based on MDRS score, and all groups showed a good response in UPDRS-III motor scores with DBS. Despite this motor response, the lowest scoring quartile group of patients (scores of 130–137) did not show improvements in quality of life (as measured with PDQ-39) compared with a control group treated with best medical therapy. Patients in the groups of higher MDRS scores (138–144) showed significant quality-of-life improvements. Given that many PD patients will be screened for DBS and denied surgery based on cognitive limitations, surgeons will sometimes be pressured by patients and families to relax the cognitive criteria. In general, however, cut-off criteria should not be relaxed because of this lack of improvement in quality of life.

Psychiatric Comorbidity

Many DBS teams include a psychiatrist or mental health professional to assist with patient screening. Neuropsychiatric issues must be addressed and stabilized prior to surgery, and new issues may emerge that require attention, such as infrequent postoperative hypomania and depression [43, 66]. Poorly treated depression, such as a score > 18 on the Beck Depression Inventory, is a contraindication to surgery. Although randomized trials have refuted an increased risk for suicide with DBS, vigilance for depression after surgery is appropriate because postoperative depression is the largest risk factor for completed suicide [50]. A previous history of impulse control disorder, prior suicide attempts, and a younger age of disease onset are risk factors for attempted suicide. Castrioto et al. [61] published an extensive review of the complex topic of behavioral effects of DBS. In brief, mood changes often follow DBS, and it can be unclear whether they are caused by medication changes, surgical trauma, or DBS therapy itself. Regardless of cause, mood changes require appropriate evaluation and treatment to preserve DBS-related quality-of-life improvements, which emphasizes the need for a team approach to patient care.

Attitudinal issues also need to be assessed during the evaluation process. Some patients are unable to "give up control" and allow for physician programming of the device. Such patients are often unable to obtain much benefit from DBS because they frequently self-alter the device programming. Patients who are unable to cooperate with the team evaluation process because of attitudinal issues should raise concerns. A patient's social environment is also a factor, as the patient must be able to make multiple follow-up appointments for programming and future battery changes.

Medical Comorbidity

Patients must be able to physically tolerate DBS lead placement surgery that involves either an awake burr-hole craniotomy or an exposure to general anesthesia. Patients also need to be able to cooperate with device programming sessions and future internal pulse generator replacement procedures. Active systemic diseases such as untreated cancer, active cardiopulmonary disease, or coagulopathy preclude DBS therapy. Rughani et al. [67] used the Nationwide Inpatient Sample (NIS) from 1999 to 2008 to review acute complications occurring in 4145 patients with PD who underwent movement disorder surgery, primarily DBS. The presence of more than one medical comorbidity was associated with an elevated risk of both in-hospital complications and mortality. The risk of either remained low, however, at 5 and 0.5%, respectively.

Age

Currently, there is not an absolute age cut-off for consideration of DBS surgery. As with any surgery, younger patients are less likely to have significant comorbidities and are better able to recover from complications such as pneumonia or deep venous thrombosis; however, physicians should set reasonable expectations regarding expected outcomes. Motor improvements, as measured with UPDRS-III, were greater for patients younger than 56 years old and with a shorter disease duration (less than 16 years) [68]. When patients were stratified as older or younger than 65 years of age, there was no difference in motor improvement, but the older group had a smaller improvement in the quality-of-life measures [69]. It is important to acknowledge that while age was not a specific cut-off in large prospective DBS trials showing good efficacy of both STN and GPi DBS, the average age of patients who otherwise met enrollment criteria was only ~60 years [41, 42]. The NIS review revealed an increased risk of acute complications and mortality with increasing age. Increasing age, however, was essentially a proxy for multiple medical comorbidities and was not independently associated with increased risks [67]. Given the additional risks inherent in operating on older patients, some surgeons advocate implanting unilateral leads.

Target Selection

Stimulation of the VIM thalamus improves tremor associated with PD but does not produce significant improvement in other motor symptoms. Stimulation of either the STN or GPi can be used to improve the cardinal features of the disease. Choices between the targets have generally been guided by physician preference and expertise informed by outcomes of retrospective studies. To address this limitation, three large prospective trials were undertaken that directly compare GPi DBS and STN DBS: the NIH COMPARE trial (using unilateral stimulation) [46], the VA Cooperative study (bilateral) [41, 70], and the NSTAPS trial (bilateral) [42].

Summary for the Clinician
- The successful use of DBS therapy requires careful patient selection.
- The correct clinical diagnosis of Parkinson's disease and a reproducible response to dopamine therapy are critical selection criteria.
- Disability from nonmotor symptoms and medical comorbidities must be carefully considered before offering surgery.
- STN or GPi DBS can be equally effectively employed to treat the cardinal motor symptoms.

For treatment of motor symptoms, it is important to consider which symptoms are the most disabling to the patient. For tremor, stimulation of either the GPi or STN produces profound tremor reduction, with neither target being more efficacious [42, 46]. Some physicians tend to recommend STN stimulation for patients with tremor predominance. Anecdotally, the tremor suppression with STN stimulation tends to occur more quickly and more dramatically, being observable in the operating room. This rapid tremor suppression with STN stimulation may lead to an erroneous impression of a more effective tremor control. In the treatment of rigidity, the NIH COMPARE trial showed a slight benefit of unilateral STN stimulation, but for bilateral implantation, neither target has been shown to be superior [41, 42, 46]. For bradykinesia, no randomized trial has shown an advantage of one target over the other. In 2005, Anderson et al. demonstrated a trend suggesting that bilateral STN stimulation may be more effective than GPi stimulation, but this trend was not statistically significant. The authors also showed a difference in favor of stimulation of the GPi in the improvement of dyskinesia [71], and in unilateral cases, the stimulation of the GPi also showed a trend toward inducing more improvement [46].

For nonmotor symptoms such as cognition and speech, stimulation of the GPi is believed to be superior to stimulation of the STN. Memory has been shown to decline faster in STN DBS patients [41], and while the COMPARE study showed no difference in primary outcomes of mood and cognition, more secondary cognitive issues were seen with STN targets. Speech may be more affected by STN DBS than GPi DBS. Several studies have shown reduced speech intelligibility and induced dysarthria with STN stimulation [45, 72, 73].

Medication reduction is consistently more pronounced with STN stimulation than with GPI [70, 74]. Battery drain is higher with GPI stimulation than with STN [70]. Adding these two factors together, STN stimulation is more cost-effective.

Summary

For appropriately selected patients with PD, DBS can provide profound improvements in tremor, rigidity, bradykinesia, dyskinesia, and motor fluctuations. Prospective trials show that DBS produces improvements in quality of life beyond what is achievable with best medical therapy. Stimulation of either the GPi or STN is effective. Reproducing the outcomes documented in high-quality, prospective trials, however, requires careful patient evaluation and selection through the cooperation of a multidisciplinary team. PD remains a progressive disorder, and it is important that patients and families be multiply counseled regarding realistic expectations.

References

1. de Lau LM, Breteler MM. Epidemiology of Parkinson's disease. Lancet Neurol. 2006;5(6):525–35.
2. Nussbaum RL, Ellis CE. Alzheimer's disease and Parkinson's disease. N Engl J Med. 2003;348(14):1356–64.

3. Dorsey ER, et al. Projected number of people with Parkinson disease in the most populous nations, 2005 through 2030. Neurology. 2007;68(5):384–6.
4. Gibb WR, Lees AJ. The relevance of the Lewy body to the pathogenesis of idiopathic Parkinson's disease. J Neurol Neurosurg Psychiatry. 1988;51(6):745–52.
5. Gasser T. Usefulness of genetic testing in PD and PD trials: a balanced review. J Parkinsons Dis. 2015;5:209–15.
6. Warner TT, Schapira AH. Genetic and environmental factors in the cause of Parkinson's disease. Ann Neurol. 2003;53(Suppl 3):S16–23. discussion S23–25
7. Selikhova M, et al. A clinico-pathological study of subtypes in Parkinson's disease. Brain. 2009;132(Pt 11):2947–57.
8. Thenganatt MA, Jankovic J. Parkinson disease subtypes. JAMA Neurol. 2014;71(4): 499–504.
9. Movement Disorder Society Task Force on Rating Scales for Parkinson's, Disease. The Unified Parkinson's Disease Rating Scale (UPDRS): status and recommendations. Mov Disord. 2003;18(7):738–50.
10. Jankovic J. Parkinson's disease: clinical features and diagnosis. J Neurol Neurosurg Psychiatry. 2008;79(4):368–76.
11. Hauser RA, Auinger P, Parkinson Study G. Determination of minimal clinically important change in early and advanced Parkinson's disease. Mov Disord. 2011;26(5):813–8.
12. Macleod AD, Taylor KS, Counsell CE. Mortality in Parkinson's disease: a systematic review and meta-analysis. Mov Disord. 2014;29(13):1615–22.
13. Galvan A, Wichmann T. Pathophysiology of parkinsonism. Clin Neurophysiol. 2008;119(7):1459–74.
14. Lees AJ, Tolosa E, Olanow CW. Four pioneers of L-dopa treatment: Arvid Carlsson, Oleh Hornykiewicz, George Cotzias, and Melvin Yahr. Mov Disord. 2015;30(1):19–36.
15. Olanow CW, Brundin P. Parkinson's disease and alpha synuclein: is Parkinson's disease a prion-like disorder? Mov Disord. 2013;28(1):31–40.
16. Braak H, et al. Staging of brain pathology related to sporadic Parkinson's disease. Neurobiol Aging. 2003;24(2):197–211.
17. Halliday GM, McCann H. The progression of pathology in Parkinson's disease. Ann N Y Acad Sci. 2010;1184:188–95.
18. Cedarbaum JM, et al. Effect of supplemental carbidopa on bioavailability of L-dopa. Clin Neuropharmacol. 1986;9(2):153–9.
19. Nelson MV, et al. Pharmacokinetic and pharmacodynamic modeling of L-dopa plasma concentrations and clinical effects in Parkinson's disease after Sinemet. Clin Neuropharmacol. 1989;12(2):91–7.
20. Cotzias GC, Papavasiliou PS, Gellene R. Modification of parkinsonism--chronic treatment with L-dopa. N Engl J Med. 1969;280(7):337–45.
21. Olanow CW. Levodopa: effect on cell death and the natural history of Parkinson's disease. Mov Disord. 2015;30(1):37–44.
22. Fahn S, et al. Levodopa and the progression of Parkinson's disease. N Engl J Med. 2004;351(24):2498–508.
23. Jenner P. Molecular mechanisms of L-DOPA-induced dyskinesia. Nat Rev Neurosci. 2008;9(9):665–77.
24. Ahlskog JE, Muenter MD. Frequency of levodopa-related dyskinesias and motor fluctuations as estimated from the cumulative literature. Mov Disord. 2001;16(3):448–58.
25. Cilia R, et al. The modern pre-levodopa era of Parkinson's disease: insights into motor complications from sub-Saharan Africa. Brain. 2014;137(Pt 10):2731–42.
26. Parkinson Study G. Dopamine transporter brain imaging to assess the effects of pramipexole vs levodopa on Parkinson disease progression. JAMA. 2002;287(13):1653–61.
27. Whone AL, et al. Slower progression of Parkinson's disease with ropinirole versus levodopa: the REAL-PET study. Ann Neurol. 2003;54(1):93–101.
28. American Academy of Neurology. Practice Parameter: Treatment of Parkinson Disease with Motor Fluctuations and Dyskinesia. 2006; Available from: aan.com/guidelines.

29. Olanow CW, et al. Continuous intrajejunal infusion of levodopa-carbidopa intestinal gel for patients with advanced Parkinson's disease: a randomised, controlled, double-blind, double-dummy study. Lancet Neurol. 2014;13(2):141–9.
30. Guridi J, Lozano AM. A brief history of pallidotomy. Neurosurgery. 1997;41(5):1169–80. discussion 1180-3
31. Speelman JD, Bosch DA. Resurgence of functional neurosurgery for Parkinson's disease: a historical perspective. Mov Disord. 1998;13(3):582–8.
32. DeLong MR, et al. The contribution of basal ganglia to limb control. Prog Brain Res. 1986;64:161–74.
33. Bergman H, Wichmann T, DeLong MR. Reversal of experimental parkinsonism by lesions of the subthalamic nucleus. Science. 1990;249(4975):1436–8.
34. Pollak P, et al. Effects of the stimulation of the subthalamic nucleus in Parkinson disease. Rev Neurol (Paris). 1993;149(3):175–6.
35. McCairn KW, Turner RS. Deep brain stimulation of the globus pallidus internus in the parkinsonian primate: local entrainment and suppression of low-frequency oscillations. J Neurophysiol. 2009;101(4):1941–60.
36. Brown P. Bad oscillations in Parkinson's disease. J Neural Transm Suppl. 2006;70:27–30.
37. Wingeier B, et al. Intra-operative STN DBS attenuates the prominent beta rhythm in the STN in Parkinson's disease. Exp Neurol. 2006;197(1):244–51.
38. Shimamoto SA, et al. Subthalamic nucleus neurons are synchronized to primary motor cortex local field potentials in Parkinson's disease. J Neurosci. 2013;33(17):7220–33.
39. Chiken S, Nambu A. Disrupting neuronal transmission: mechanism of DBS? Front Syst Neurosci. 2014;8:33.
40. Deuschl G, et al. A randomized trial of deep-brain stimulation for Parkinson's disease. N Engl J Med. 2006;355(9):896–908.
41. Weaver FM, et al. Randomized trial of deep brain stimulation for Parkinson disease: thirty-six-month outcomes. Neurology. 2012;79(1):55–65.
42. Odekerken VJ, et al. Subthalamic nucleus versus globus pallidus bilateral deep brain stimulation for advanced Parkinson's disease (NSTAPS study): a randomised controlled trial. Lancet Neurol. 2013;12(1):37–44.
43. Krack P, et al. Five-year follow-up of bilateral stimulation of the subthalamic nucleus in advanced Parkinson's disease. N Engl J Med. 2003;349(20):1925–34.
44. Hamani C, et al. Bilateral subthalamic nucleus stimulation for Parkinson's disease: a systematic review of the clinical literature. Neurosurgery. 2005;56(6):1313–21. discussion 1321-4
45. Kleiner-Fisman G, et al. Subthalamic nucleus deep brain stimulation: summary and meta-analysis of outcomes. Mov Disord. 2006;21(Suppl 14):S290–304.
46. Okun MS, et al. Cognition and mood in Parkinson's disease in subthalamic nucleus versus globus pallidus interna deep brain stimulation: the COMPARE trial. Ann Neurol. 2009;65(5):586–95.
47. Limousin P, et al. Multicentre European study of thalamic stimulation in parkinsonian and essential tremor. J Neurol Neurosurg Psychiatry. 1999;66(3):289–96.
48. Aviles-Olmos I, et al. Long-term outcome of subthalamic nucleus deep brain stimulation for Parkinson's disease using an MRI-guided and MRI-verified approach. J Neurol Neurosurg Psychiatry. 2014;85(12):1419–25.
49. Funkiewiez A, et al. Long term effects of bilateral subthalamic nucleus stimulation on cognitive function, mood, and behaviour in Parkinson's disease. J Neurol Neurosurg Psychiatry. 2004;75(6):834–9.
50. Weintraub D, et al. Suicide ideation and behaviours after STN and GPi DBS surgery for Parkinson's disease: results from a randomised, controlled trial. J Neurol Neurosurg Psychiatry. 2013;84(10):1113–8.
51. Weintraub D, et al. Clinical spectrum of impulse control disorders in Parkinson's disease. Mov Disord. 2015;30(2):121–7.
52. Tarsy D, et al. Progression of Parkinson's disease following thalamic deep brain stimulation for tremor. Stereotact Funct Neurosurg. 2005;83(5–6):222–7.

53. Bang Henriksen, M., et al., Surviving 10 years with deep brain stimulation for Parkinson's disease - a follow-up of 79 patients. Eur J Neurol, 2014. (in press).
54. Okun MS, et al. Management of referred deep brain stimulation failures: a retrospective analysis from 2 movement disorders centers. Arch Neurol. 2005;62(8):1250–5.
55. Verstraeten A, Theuns J, Van Broeckhoven C. Progress in unraveling the genetic etiology of Parkinson disease in a genomic era. Trends Genet. 2015;31(3):140–9.
56. Hughes AJ, et al. Accuracy of clinical diagnosis of idiopathic Parkinson's disease: a clinico-pathological study of 100 cases. J Neurol Neurosurg Psychiatry. 1992;55(3):181–4.
57. Schuepbach WM, et al. Neurostimulation for Parkinson's disease with early motor complications. N Engl J Med. 2013;368(7):610–22.
58. Mestre TA, et al. Subthalamic nucleus-deep brain stimulation for early motor complications in Parkinson's disease-the EARLYSTIM trial: early is not always better. Mov Disord. 2014;29(14):1751–6.
59. Hoehn MM, Yahr MD. Parkinsonism: onset, progression and mortality. Neurology. 1967;17(5):427–42.
60. Bronstein JM, et al. Deep brain stimulation for Parkinson disease: an expert consensus and review of key issues. Arch Neurol. 2011;68(2):165.
61. Castrioto A, et al. Mood and behavioural effects of subthalamic stimulation in Parkinson's disease. Lancet Neurol. 2014;13(3):287–305.
62. Massano J, Garrett C. Deep brain stimulation and cognitive decline in Parkinson's disease: a clinical review. Front Neurol. 2012;3:66.
63. Lang AE, et al. Deep brain stimulation: preoperative issues. Mov Disord. 2006;21(Suppl 14):S171–96.
64. Llebaria G, et al. Cut-off score of the Mattis dementia rating scale for screening dementia in Parkinson's disease. Mov Disord. 2008;23(11):1546–50.
65. Witt K, et al. Negative impact of borderline global cognitive scores on quality of life after subthalamic nucleus stimulation in Parkinson's disease. J Neurol Sci. 2011;310(1–2):261–6.
66. Daniele A, et al. Cognitive and behavioural effects of chronic stimulation of the sub-thalamic nucleus in patients with Parkinson's disease. J Neurol Neurosurg Psychiatry. 2003;74(2):175–82.
67. Rughani AI, Hodaie M, Lozano AM. Acute complications of movement disorders surgery: effects of age and comorbidities. Mov Disord. 2013;28(12):1661–7.
68. Welter ML, et al. Clinical predictive factors of subthalamic stimulation in Parkinson's disease. Brain. 2002;125(Pt 3):575–83.
69. Derost PP, et al. Is DBS-STN appropriate to treat severe Parkinson disease in an elderly population? Neurology. 2007;68(17):1345–55.
70. Follett KA, et al. Pallidal versus subthalamic deep-brain stimulation for Parkinson's disease. N Engl J Med. 2010;362(22):2077–91.
71. Anderson VC, et al. Pallidal vs subthalamic nucleus deep brain stimulation in Parkinson disease. Arch Neurol. 2005;62(4):554–60.
72. Hartinger M, et al. Effects of medication and subthalamic nucleus deep brain stimulation on tongue movements in speakers with Parkinson's disease using electropalatography: a pilot study. Clin Linguist Phon. 2011;25(3):210–30.
73. Putzer M, Barry WJ, Moringlane JR. Effect of bilateral stimulation of the subthalamic nucleus on different speech subsystems in patients with Parkinson's disease. Clin Linguist Phon. 2008;22(12):957–73.
74. Krack P, Hariz MI. Deep brain stimulation in Parkinson's disease: reconciliation of evidence-based medicine with clinical practice. Lancet Neurol. 2013;12(1):25–6.

Subthalamic Nucleus Deep Brain Stimulation with Microelectrode Recording Using a Frame

2

Andres L. Maldonado-Naranjo, Andre G. Machado, Michal Gostkowski, Hubert H. Fernandez, and Sean J. Nagel

- The most common site for electrode implantation in patients diagnosed with PD is the STN.
- Patients with a diagnosis of idiopathic PD based on clinical examination, response to levodopa, and disease progression are candidates for surgical evaluation.
- A volumetric, gadolinium-enhanced, 3 tesla MRI is used for presurgical planning although the reliability of 7 tesla MRI is under study.
- We currently use a combination of direct and indirect methods to target the subthalamic nucleus.
- The most effective site for stimulation is thought to be the dorsolateral portion of the STN which corresponds with the sensorimotor region of the nucleus.
- An intraoperative 0-arm study and microelectrode recording data are used to interpolate the relative location of the electrode to the STN.
- We usually position the most ventral contact (the one near the tip of the DBS lead), at the ventral STN. As we gradually increase the amplitude during testing of the macroelectrode, improvements in tremor, bradykinesia, and rigidity are expected.

A. L. Maldonado-Naranjo
Department of Neurosurgery, Cleveland Clinic, Neurologic Institute, Cleveland, OH, USA

A. G. Machado · S. J. Nagel (✉)
Department of Neurosurgery, Cleveland Clinic, Neurologic Institute, Cleveland, OH, USA

Cleveland Clinic, Neurologic Institute, Center for Neurological Restoration, Cleveland, OH, USA

M. Gostkowski · H. H. Fernandez
Cleveland Clinic, Neurologic Institute, Center for Neurological Restoration, Cleveland, OH, USA

Department of Neurology, Cleveland Clinic, Neurologic Institute, Cleveland, OH, USA

© Springer Nature Switzerland AG 2019
R. R. Goodman (ed.), *Surgery for Parkinson's Disease*,
https://doi.org/10.1007/978-3-319-23693-3_2

Introduction

The first attempts to surgically treat Parkinson's disease (PD) beginning in the 1930s predated the discovery of the medications that would eventually derail its further development [1]. These procedures, now abandoned, often focused on ablating the central nervous system at different sites including the posterior roots, anterolateral column, lateral pyramidal track, and precentral gyrus. Injection of procaine into the sensory nerves was also considered [2, 3]. These earliest attempts yielded partial or no benefit but were hampered even more by the significant morbidity of the operations.

Irving Cooper, while performing a pedunculotomy in a patient with tremor, inadvertently ligated the anterior choroidal artery. The patient awoke to find his tremor and rigidity resolved [4]. While ligation of the choroidal artery may on occasion improve the symptoms of PD, when the infarction was confined to the globus pallidus, the variation in the vascular territory often led to infarctions of the internal capsule or thalamus that consequently resulted in hemiparesis or other neurological deficits. Spiegel and Wycis developed the first stereotactic frame for human use and played a major role in advancing the surgical treatment of movement disorders [5, 6]. Interest in surgery, except for a few centers, waned after L-dopa was introduced in the late 1960s and did not re-emerge until the 1980s when Benabid (1987), while performing thalamotomy, noted that electrical stimulation, intended to avoid injuring functional sites, induced a reversible improvement of tremor [7]. These findings were the basis for his study of chronic ventral intermediate thalamic electrical stimulation in 33 patients with tremor [8]. His group later reported the first case of subthalamic nucleus (STN) deep brain stimulation in PD [9]. Although the internal globus pallidus (GPi) and the ventral thalamus (VT) are also targeted, the most common site for electrode implantation, as a treatment for PD, remains the STN. While the debate remains on the merits of STN versus globus pallidus stimulation in PD, a recent meta-analysis showed quantitative evidence for significant improvement of patient's symptoms, functionality, and quality of life, after STN DBS [10] (Fig. 2.1).

Patient Selection

At the Cleveland Clinic's Center for Neurological Restoration, potential surgical candidates are evaluated by a movement disorders neurologist, specialized movement disorder nurse or physician assistant, neurosurgeon, neuropsychologist, and in most cases by a movement disorder psychiatrist. Under some circumstances, a bioethics assessment is requested. Testing also includes motor testing in the "on" and "off" states with video recording and brain MRI with gadolinium. Patients are then discussed thoroughly in a multidisciplinary conference weighing the risk versus benefit of DBS, evaluating the most ideal target and method (e.g., unilateral versus bilateral; staged versus simultaneous). A recent study by our group found that 27.3% of patients referred to our center were not offered DBS. The most common

Fig. 2.1 Axial sequence 7 T MRI (top) and 3 T MRI T2 (bottom) merged with volumetric study depicting the subthalamic nucleus and red nucleus

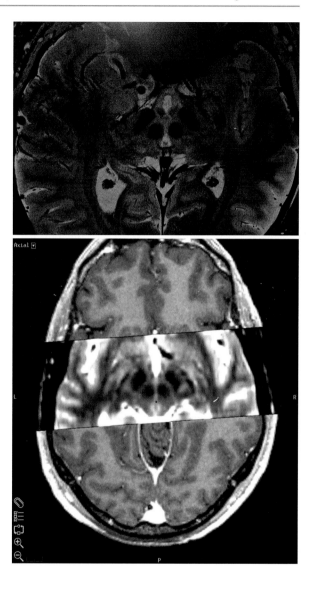

reasons for exclusion were cognitive impairment (32%), early PD or non-optimized medical therapy (29.5%), behavioral issues (21.3%), likely diagnosis of secondary parkinsonism or atypical parkinsonism (13.1%), poor levodopa response (11.4%), unrealistic patient's perception of surgical goals (9.8%), predominant axial symptoms (6.5%), significant medical or surgical comorbidities (6.5%), and abnormal brain imaging (3.2%). Of the excluded patients, 29.5% had multiple exclusion factors, most commonly with the combination of cognitive and behavioral dysfunction [11]. Except in unusual circumstances, only patients with a clear diagnosis of idiopathic PD based on clinical examination, response to levodopa and disease progression, proceed with surgical evaluation. To date, patients with atypical parkinsonian syndromes, such as dementia with Lewy bodies, vascular parkinsonism, or other parkinsonian-plus syndromes, have not shown a favorable response to DBS. Clinicians look for symptoms that are likely to benefit the most from DBS. STN DBS most consistently improves the classic dopa-responsive motor symptoms of PD, such as bradykinesia and rigidity, and in addition also relieves medication-resistant resting tremor [12].

Since DBS tends to mirror the effect of levodopa on time, patients who do not improve with levodopa are also unlikely to improve with DBS. The degree of improvement following administration of dopaminergic agents is conventionally tested using the motor subscale of the Unified Parkinson Disease Rating Scale (UPDRS-III). An improvement of approximately 33% in the UPDRS-III score in the on state with a minimum UPDRS-III score of 30 (out of total possible 108) in the off state are useful benchmarks [13]. Off medication, motor symptoms have been shown to improve the UPDRS score by 40–60%. On the other hand, non-motor features of PD, such as impaired cognitive function and dysautonomia, do not respond to DBS. In patients who are significantly disabled by the motor features of the disease, but who show minimal or no change in cognition, the risks of DBS may be offset by the estimated benefit.

Unfortunately, cognitive decline, including dementia, is a frequent finding in patients with advancing PD and DBS that can significantly worsen cognition, particularly among at-risk patients. A Mini-Mental Status Examination (MMSE) score of equal to or less than 24 has been proposed as a simple screening criterion for exclusion [13]. However, we prefer a full neuropsychological evaluation completed by psychologists who are active participants in the DBS program. Because many patients who may significantly benefit from DBS from a motor standpoint also have some cognitive impairment, we assess patients "holistically," attempting to best estimate the risk and likely magnitude of cognitive decline, along with the potential benefits of surgery. Patients with mood disorders, particularly severe depression and anxiety or psychosis that are refractory to treatment, are often excluded as surgical candidates. Older patients with PD can be at higher risk for worse outcomes [14]. However, for many older patients with significant motor symptoms and adverse levodopa effects, in good health, without dementia or psychiatric problems, surgery is still often a good choice and they can experience significant improvements in quality of life. Claustrophobia is a significant problem for patients undergoing DBS guided by microelectrode recording (MER) with a stereotactic head frame, as this condition could manifest during the awake intraoperative testing, limiting the utility of the MER and increasing the risk for lead misplacement.

Patients with significant bilateral symptoms benefit from bilateral DBS. Patients with bilateral symptoms who undergo unilateral DBS often do not benefit fully from surgery and many present significant challenges in management, postoperatively. Previous ablative surgery is not an absolute exclusion. For instance, a patient with previous unilateral pallidotomy might seek treatment to control symptoms on the opposite site. Alternatively, a patient with a suboptimal outcome following a previous pallidotomy might further benefit from STN DBS [15]. A summary of the inclusion and exclusion criteria is found in Table 2.1.

Table 2.1 Inclusion and exclusion criteria for STN DBS

Inclusion criteria	Exclusion criteria	Concerns
Confirmed diagnosis of idiopathic Parkinson's disease	Secondary parkinsonism or atypical parkinsonism	Coagulopathy, antiplatelet, or anticoagulant use
PD with significant or disabling motor symptoms	Suboptimal Parkinson's disease medical treatment	Prior cranial surgery
Dyskinesia and other drug-related side effects, and potential to decreased dosage post-DBS	Cognitive impairment, dementia	Advanced age
Improvement of UPDRS-III score of >33%, or a minimum UPDRS-III score of 30/108 in the off state	Poor levodopa response	Medical comorbidities, including cardiac, lung, and uncontrolled hypertension
Appropriate expectations from surgery and understanding of outcomes	Unrealistic patient's perception of surgical goals	Increased risk for infection in patients with primary or secondary immunodeficiency
No structural lesions on imaging studies	Depression, anxiety, psychosis, claustrophobia	Structural lesions or findings that could interfere with electrode implantation

Preoperative Evaluation

In addition to the standard preoperative surgical testing and evaluation, special attention is focused on select medical comorbidities, in patients scheduled for DBS with MER. Uncontrolled hypertension perioperatively likely contributes to the risk of intraoperative bleeding, the most significant complication of DBS. Estimates vary but the risk is reported to be between 1.5% and 3%, with a risk of permanent morbidity of 0.5 and 1% [16–18]. We prefer a systolic blood pressure of equal to or less than 130 mmHg intraoperatively, which is then slowly liberalized during the postoperative period.

Antiplatelet and anticoagulation medications, as well as nonsteroidal anti-inflammatory medications, are stopped 7–10 days before the surgery or a warfarin-to-heparin bridge is initiated, in high-risk individuals. The risks of stopping anticoagulation therefore should be carefully weighed against the potential benefit of DBS surgery. In general, we favor consultation with cardiology or cerebrovascular neurology to clarify the risk to the patient, of medication cessation.

Patients with an increased risk of developing infections, such as patients with diabetes and chronic steroid use, are advised of the elevated risks. In addition, patients with history of poor wound healing or loss of elasticity in the skin may be at increased risk for hardware erosion. Finally, post-DBS, patients should avoid large magnetic fields. A limited number of MRI sequences are compatible with DBS systems, under strict guidelines. Therefore, patients requiring frequent imaging with MRI might not be appropriate candidates [19–21].

Imaging

In our center, we obtain a volumetric MRI, gadolinium-enhanced, with T1- and T2-weighted images, several days or weeks prior to surgery. In general, we feel that patients with an MRI older than 2–3 months should undergo new imaging, to rule out subclinical changes that may influence planning, such as small lacunar strokes or other intracranial lesions. T2 and inversion recovery images are beneficial for direct targeting of STN. Reducing motion artifact due to tremor or dyskinesia is challenging in some patients. We continue to use a 3 Tesla MRI for planning; however, with the introduction of 7 Tesla MRI, we expect this will replace the 3 T as our imaging modality of choice for some patients. Whether clinically significant distortion is evident on 7 T MRIs is still under study. Motion artifact is compounded in 7 T machines and may limit their use in some patients. A study recently found significant correlation between identical targets in central parts of the brain when using 7 Tesla MRI as compared to 1.5 Tesla MRI [22]. Ongoing studies are being performed in our center to assess the reliability of 7 Tesla MRI as a tool for preoperative planning in our patients.

When MRI is contraindicated, CT is used for planning. Although CT lacks the resolution of an MRI, it is not susceptible to the distortional artifact produced by inhomogeneity in the magnetic field and thus more accurately represents the actual position of the intracerebral structures. However, in CT scans, the commissures are less clearly identifiable and the STN cannot be visualized, so surgical planning is performed exclusively by indirect targeting, with greater reliance on intraoperative microelectrode and macroelectrode physiology.

Targeting

Targeting can be performed prior to the day of the procedure or on the morning of surgery. We currently use a combination of direct and indirect targeting. Direct targeting is based on direct visualization of the STN on MRI sequences such as T2, proton density, and inversion recovery [23]. The STN lies anterior and lateral to the more easily visualized red nucleus. The anterior border of the red nucleus can be used as a landmark for identifying the posterior and inferior margin of the STN. While the goal of surgery is to place DBS electrodes in the motor territory of the STN, in the dorsolateral compartment of the nucleus, at a distance of about 2 mm from the internal capsule, the tip of the electrode is often placed posteriorly and inferiorly in the nucleus in such a fashion as to position the upper contacts of the quadripolar leads in the desired territory (Fig. 2.2).

Indirect targeting is based on internal landmarks such as the midcommissural point (MCP), the midpoint of the AC-PC (anterior-posterior commissure) line. The coordinates we often use to initiate targeting for the STN are 10 to 13 mm lateral to the midline, 4–5 mm ventral to the intercomissural plane, and 3–4 mm posterior to the MCP.

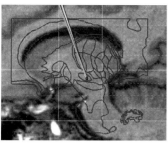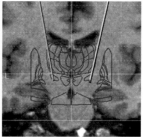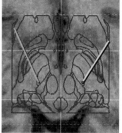

Fig. 2.2 Sagittal, coronal, and axial views demonstrating subthalamic nucleus target selection in the dorsolateral region

There are several strategies for selecting an entry point. We start at the intersection of the coronal suture and the middle frontal gyrus and adjust anteriorly as needed. A more posterior entry point is used on occasion, but risks injuring the precentral gyrus. As most patients with PD will have evidence of some age-related atrophy, a more medial entry point through the superior frontal gyrus often traverses the ventricle. Going through the ventricle is a choice in stereotactic neurosurgery, and some centers may routinely select transventricular approaches. In some of the emerging DBS indications, a transventricular route is often the best choice for reaching the desired target [24]. However, when STN is the desired target, a trajectory that avoids the ventricle effectively eliminates the risk of intraventricular hemorrhage and may reduce the incidence of postoperative confusion [25]. The entry point and trajectory are generally planned to avoid vascular structures as well as sulci. A typical trajectory would transverse the anterior thalamus, zona incerta, STN and the substantia nigra (SN), after passing through the crown of a gyrus. The trajectory can be visualized with orthogonal axial, coronal, and sagittal views, as well as with a "probe's eye" view, advancing millimeter by millimeter along the trajectory to look for anatomical structures that will be along the path of the cannula and electrodes (Fig. 2.3).

Frame Placement

Patients are typically admitted to the hospital the night before surgery with their PD medications held. Surgery is then performed in the "off state," to enhance the neurophysiological recordings and measure symptoms with stimulation. Oral hypoglycemic agents are also discontinued, whereas the morning dose of an antihypertensive medication should be given before surgery. Some authors recommend beta-blockers be stopped before surgery, due to potential reversible changes in STN activity [26]. However, we have not incorporated this into our practice and often utilize beta-blockers to manage blood pressure intraoperatively.

Stereotactic frames used for DBS include the CRW, Riechert-Mundinger, and Leksell. Each frame has been extensively tested for targeting errors [27]. Accuracy

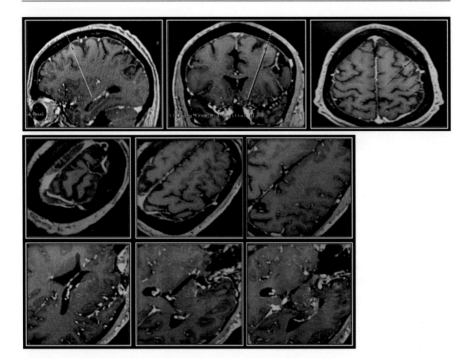

Fig. 2.3 Top panel: Sagittal, coronal, and axial views showing a proposed trajectory. This entry point is at the middle frontal gyrus and in this example the trajectory is lateral to the ventricle. Bottom panel: Probes eye view of the same trajectory

is inversely related to the targeting error. In phantom models, the Leksell system, CRW, and STarFix have targeting errors of 1.7, 1.8, and 0.42 mm, respectively. Taking into consideration brain shift, in the clinical setting, targeting errors are 2.78 mm (SD 0.25) for NexFrame, 2.65 mm (SD 0.22) for the CRW and 1.99 mm (SD 0.92) for the STarFix. Our preference is to use the Leksell frame for DBS with MER; however, this is largely based on familiarity, availability, and cost and not a belief that this is a superior frame.

On the morning of surgery, the patient's hair is clipped and pin points are prepared with betadine. We use lidocaine and marcaine mixture, without epinephrine, for local anesthesia. The base of the frame is placed parallel to a line extending from the lateral canthus or orbital floor to the tragus in order to parallel the AC-PC plane. The head should be centered in the midline of the frame. The frame base should not be in contact with the skin, to avoid development of pressure ulcers. The pins are finger tightened until the outer layer of the bone is purchased. Over tightening of the pins can distort the frame and lower the accuracy of the system. We usually will place the frame in the operating room, under sedation.

Once the frame is in place, the patient undergoes a stereo head CT scan. Several image-guiding systems are available for merging and target/trajectory planning. We use the Stealth Station s7 (Medtronic, Minneapolis) for stereotactic planning.

Patient Positioning and Anesthesia

The patient is positioned supine on the operating table. Sequential compression devices, if used, should be removed at the time of intraoperative testing. The frame is fixed to the operating table with an adapter and the head/neck positioned for patient comfort. Sedation is started with propofol. Invasive arterial blood pressure monitoring is initiated, if the blood pressure is labile. Our anesthesiology team often utilizes hydralazine, labetalol, and nicardipine for intraoperative blood pressure control. Preoperative antibiotics should be given 30 min before incision. We pre-wash the scalp for 7 min with Hibiclens solution, followed by application of an alcohol-based solution. A Foley catheter is inserted once sedation has started. An intraoperative imaging system (O-arm, Surgical Imaging System, Medtronic) is brought into the field and aligned in parallel with the frame base (Fig. 2.4). The rings are positioned on the frame, and the y and z coordinates are set and independently confirmed by an assistant.

We use a disposable, waterproof, DBS-specific plastic drape with an Ioban center. The outer borders of the drape are affixed to the O-arm to accommodate table adjustment during the procedure. One important detail is to leave enough slack in

Fig. 2.4 Intraoperative setup with O-arm draped into the field

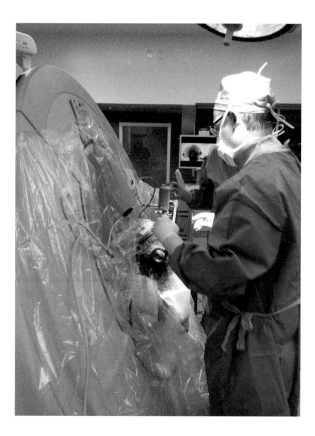

the draping to accommodate movement of the O-arm during the procedure. All cables, suction, and bipolar are connected to the drape itself for surgeon's easy access. The stereotactic arc is attached to the Leksell frame, the x coordinate set, and the ring angle adjusted. The site of the entry point is marked on the Ioban covered skin after the angle is identified. A linear or curvilinear incision is planned around the entry point.

The surgical site is infiltrated with lidocaine and we also infiltrate local anesthetic along the planned subgaleal tunneling path, posterior to the incision. A self-retaining retractor is positioned after hemostasis of the scalp and galea. The cannula is used to mark the point of entry on the skull. A 14-mm pneumatic drill perforates the skull to expose the dura and the remnants of the internal table are removed with a curette and bone bleeding plugged with bone wax. The inner table is undermined with a Kerrison if it is evident that the cannula will deflect off of the bone on entry. The anchoring device (Stim-Loc Anchoring device, Medtronic) is secured to the skull by using 4 mm screws. The clip is deployed to verify it will lock and then removed. The dura mater is coagulated, opened in a cruciate fashion, and its leaflets retracted with bipolar cauterization over the entry point. A small corticectomy is performed by coagulation of the pia and incision with an 11 blade. Careful entry point planning will minimize the likelihood of a cortical vessel being in the field. Nonetheless, mobilization of a cortical vessel is sometimes the only option.

The anesthesia team is then asked to arrest sedation and awaken the patient. A microdrive is assembled and a premeasured cannula with a stylet insert is advanced 15 mm dorsal to the target in the preparation for MER. Gelfoam and fibrin glue are placed in the burr hole around the cannula to minimize CSF loss and pneumocephalus.

Microelectrode Recording

The STN is an obliquely oriented oval-shaped structure between 125 and 238 mm3 in volume. We start our MER at 15 mm dorsal to the target. As the microelectrode is advanced, the anterior thalamus or reticular thalamus is entered. Relative quiescence is recorded, as the electrode passes through zona incerta (ZI). A larger gap (thicker ZI) between the thalamus and STN is noted, if the trajectory is more anterior. The anterior thalamic nuclei have low density and slow firing rates, interposed with bursting cells that spike at a rate of about 15 Hz [28]. Compared to the other regions, the ZI is relatively silent, with occasional large-amplitude neurons or bursting neurons with rates between 25 and 40 Hz [29]. The dorsal border of STN is remarkable for its usually distinct and sudden increase in background noise, followed by isolation of the first STN cells.

On entering the STN, a pattern of tonic, irregular neuronal firing emerges with rates between 30 and 50 Hz and frequent multiunit recordings [30]. This spike rate is significantly higher than observed in a non-parkinsonian state [31]. Occasionally, a second neuronal type that shows synchronized bursting with the patient's tremor is observed. When neuronal units are well isolated, we check for kinesthetic driving by passively moving the joints on the opposite side of the body. We examine for upper and lower extremity passive joint movement as well as active movement of the jaw and tongue. When clear kinesthetic driving is identified, it corroborates a trajectory through the motor territory of the STN. While the somatotopy of the STN is not as organized as in the cortex or ventral posterior thalamic nuclei, the bulk of cells corresponding to the upper extremity are positioned more laterally than the leg cells [31]. The most effective site for stimulation is thought to be the dorsolateral portion of the STN, which corresponds with the sensorimotor region of the nucleus [32]. A microelectrode track that records from 4–6 mm in the STN, with strong kinesthetic driving, and does not elicit "capsular" effects at low amplitudes, is usually indicative of a trajectory in which the DBS lead should be implanted. However, many centers prefer to record multiple MER trajectories through the STN, in order to better understand the three-dimensional anatomy of the subthalamic area in each patient. This needs to be weighed against the risks and disadvantages of repeated MER penetrations, including hemorrhage. After the electrode exits the STN, there is brief reduction in background noise before the SNr is entered. The pattern of activity is very distinct from that of the STN, with less modulation of activity and a constant, tonic firing rate around 50–70 Hz [28, 29, 33]. We routinely perform microstimulation between 10 and 100 microamperes along the trajectory, while looking for possible effects such as brief improvements in tremor, motor contractions suggestive of stimulation of internal capsule fibers, and oculomotor changes.

After the initial MER track, we routinely acquire an intraoperative O-arm image and use this information in combination with the physiological findings. This sequence is fused with the MRI plan and the distance between the preplanned target and the electrode tip is measured, to ascertain the error between the actual and intended location. Together with the MER data, we are then able to interpolate the relative location of the electrode to the STN. This additional data point is used to refine the target of subsequent MER tracks or macroelectrode insertion and is felt to reduce the number of penetrations required for successful localization (Fig. 2.5).

DBS Electrode Implantation and Testing

At the time of this writing there are currently two DBS lead/electrode models commercially available in the United States, each with four contacts, 1.5 mm in length and 1.27 mm in diameter. The space between contacts is 1.5 mm in the 3387 lead (Medtronic, Minneapolis) and 0.5 mm in the 3389 lead (Medtronic, Minneapolis). After the coordinates for the final target are selected, the microelectrode and cannula are removed, the frame coordinates are adjusted, and the cannula and DBS lead/macroelectrode are inserted and advanced to the target. The lead is advanced beyond the end of the cannula based on the findings from MER. We usually position the ventral-most contact, that is near the tip of the DBS lead, at the ventral STN. In many patients, a microlesional effect is observed before the stimulation is even turned on. This is manifested as reduction in motor symptoms on the contralateral hemibody.

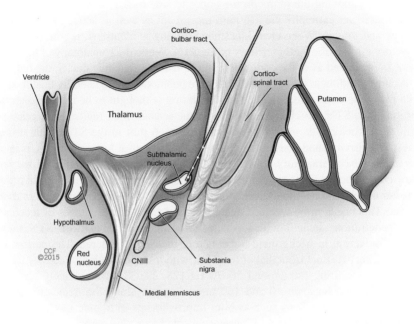

Fig. 2.5 Sample macroelectrode trajectory through the subthalamic nucleus and relationship to other regional structures

There are several options for macrostimulation settings. Our routine is to adjust the first stimulation tests to a pulse width of 90 microseconds and a rate of 130 Hz. A monopolar configuration, starting at contact 0, is tested first before moving on to the other contacts as needed. Bipolar configuration is also sometimes used. The voltage is increased progressively and the effects observed. Paresthesias that abate quickly indicate a more posterior location, but are not a contraindication for permanent implantation. As we gradually increase the amplitude, improvements in tremor, bradykinesia, and rigidity are expected. We also observe for possible side effects, such as motor contractions, diplopia, speech changes, oculomotor changes, and subjective effects such as dizziness or light-headedness. In general, we expect that the amplitude needed to cause a side effect (i.e., threshold) will be at least 50% greater than the amplitude required to control tremor and significantly improve rigidity and/or bradykinesia. If the side effects occur at a low voltage or at an amplitude similar to that required for desired effects, we consider repositioning of the lead as optimal postoperative programming may not be viable. When repositioning an electrode is required, it is recommended to move the target by a minimum of 2 mm increments, to avoid falling in the same tract from the previous lead trajectory.

Once the STN DBS electrode is satisfactorily placed, the guide tube is removed and the electrode secured with the clip. The guide wire is removed along with the carrier and microdrive. The Stim-Loc device (Medtronic, Minneapolis) is clipped, and the cap is secured after the lead is positioned in the groove of the Stim-Loc. The proximal lead is inserted into a protective casing and housed in a silastic boot fitted with two sutures. It is tunneled under the galea to the parietal boss on the ipsilateral side in order to facilitate the second part of the procedure. The excess cable is then coiled around the burr hole.

Closure and Postoperative Care

The patient is re-sedated for wound closure. The wound is irrigated and hemostasis carried out. The galea is sutured with vicryl, and special care is taken to avoid puncturing the insulation encasing the electrodes. The frame is removed, and the patient is awoken and transported to the post-anesthesia recovery unit. We routinely obtain a CT scan to rule out subclinical intracranial complications, such as an asymptomatic bleed or inadvertent electrode migration. If the CT is as expected, we liberalize the blood pressure and send the patient to a regular nursing floor room. If patients have labile blood pressure, they are admitted to a monitored bed. The majority of patients are routinely discharged after an overnight stay.

Implanting the Pulse Generator

At our institution, we implant the pulse generator 7–10 days after the lead is placed. Patients are regularly discharged on the day of surgery. Patients receive general anesthesia and are positioned with their head turned, exposing the distal end of the DBS lead. An incision approximately 2 cm inferior to clavicle and lateral to the sternum is marked on the chest. A subcutaneous pocket is created to fit the pulse generator, typically superficial to the pectoralis fascia. In thin patients, we create a pocket under the fascia of the pectoralis muscle. Of note, if a rechargeable unit is to be implanted, it is recommended that it should not be placed deeper than 1 cm from the surface in order to allow for good interaction with the recharging apparatus.

A small incision in the parieto-occipital region is made over the extension connector. From this incision, a tunneler is passed beneath the skin and externalized in the subclavicular incision. The extension wire cable is affixed to the tunneler and pulled up to the cranial incision. It is inserted into the battery and connected to the DBS lead. The incisions are irrigated and closed.

Bibliography

1. Schiefer TK, Matsumoto JY, Lee KH. Moving forward: advances in the treatment of movement disorders with deep brain stimulation. Front Integr Neurosci. 2011;5:69.
2. Bucy PC. Cortical extirpation in the treatment of involuntary movements. Am J Surg. 1948 Jan;75(1):257–63.

3. Putnam T. Relief from unilateral paralysis agitans by section of the lateral pyramidal tract. Arch Neurol Psychiatr. 1938;40:1049.
4. Cooper IS. Anterior chorodial artery ligation for involuntary movements. Science. 1953;118(3059):193.
5. Cooper IS. An investigation of neurosurgical alleviation of parkinsonism, chorea, athetosis and dystonia. Ann Intern Med. 1956;45(3):381–92.
6. Spiegel EA, Wycis HT, Marks M, Lee AJ. Stereotaxic apparatus for operations on the human brain. Science. 1947;106(2754):349–50.
7. Benabid AL, Pollak P, Louveau A, Henry S, de Rougemont J. Combined (thalamotomy and stimulation) stereotactic surgery of the VIM thalamic nucleus for bilateral Parkinson disease. Appl Neurophysiol. 1987;50(1–6):344–6.
8. Benabid AL, Pollak P, Gervason C, Hoffmann D, Gao DM, Hommel M, Perret JE, de Rougemont J. Long-term suppression of tremor by chronic stimulation of the ventral intermediate thalamic nucleus. Lancet. 1991;337(8738):403–6.
9. Benabid AL, Pollak P, Gross C, Hoffmann D, Benazzouz A, Gao DM, et al. Acute and long-term effects of subthalamic nucleus stimulation in Parkinson's disease. Stereotact Funct Neurosurg. 1994;62(1–4):76–84.
10. Perestelo-Perez L, Rivero-Santana A, Perez-Ramos J, Serrano-Perez P, Panetta J, Hilarion P. Deep brain stimulation in Parkinson's disease: meta-analysis of randomized controlled trials. J Neurol. 2014 Nov;261(11):2051–60.
11. Abboud H, Floden D, Thompson NR, Genc G, Oravivattanakul S, Alsallom F, et al. Impact of mild cognitive impairment on outcome following deep brain stimulation surgery for Parkinson's disease. Parkinsonism Relat Disord. 2015 Mar;21(3):249–53.
12. Weaver F, Follett K, Hur K, Ippolito D, Stern M. Deep brain stimulation in Parkinson disease: a metaanalysis of patient outcomes. J Neurosurg. 2005 Dec;103(6):956–67.
13. Pollak P. Deep brain stimulation for Parkinson's disease - patient selection. Handb Clin Neurol. 2013;116:97–105.
14. Saint-Cyr JA, Trepanier LL, Kumar R, Lozano AM, Lang AE. Neuropsychological consequences of chronic bilateral stimulation of the subthalamic nucleus in Parkinson's disease. Brain. 2000;123(Pt 10):2091–108.
15. Mogilner AY, Sterio D, Rezai AR, Zonenshayn M, Kelly PJ, Beric A. Subthalamic nucleus stimulation in patients with a prior pallidotomy. J Neurosurg. 2002 Apr;96(4):660–5.
16. Beric A, Kelly PJ, Rezai A, Sterio D, Mogilner A, Zonenshayn M, et al. Complications of deep brain stimulation surgery. Stereotact Funct Neurosurg. 2001;77(1–4):73–8.
17. Hariz MI. Complications of deep brain stimulation surgery. Mov Disord. 2002;17(Suppl 3):S162–6.
18. Umemura A, Jaggi JL, Hurtig HI, Siderowf AD, Colcher A, Stern MB, et al. Deep brain stimulation for movement disorders: morbidity and mortality in 109 patients. J Neurosurg. 2003 Apr;98(4):779–84.
19. Sharan A, Rezai AR, Nyenhuis JA, Hrdlicka G, Tkach J, Baker K, et al. MR safety in patients with implanted deep brain stimulation systems (DBS). Acta Neurochir Suppl. 2003;87:141–5.
20. Rezai AR, Phillips M, Baker KB, Sharan AD, Nyenhuis J, Tkach J, et al. Neurostimulation system used for deep brain stimulation (DBS): MR safety issues and implications of failing to follow safety recommendations. Investig Radiol. 2004 May;39(5):300–3.
21. Baker KB, Tkach JA, Nyenhuis JA, Phillips M, Shellock FG, Gonzalez-Martinez J, et al. Evaluation of specific absorption rate as a dosimeter of MRI-related implant heating. J Magn Reson Imaging. 2004 Aug;20(2):315–20.
22. Duchin Y, Abosch A, Yacoub E, Sapiro G, Harel N. Feasibility of using ultra-high field (7 T) MRI for clinical surgical targeting. PLoS One. 2012;7(5):e37328.
23. Andrade-Souza YM, Schwalb JM, Hamani C, Eltahawy H, Hoque T, Saint-Cyr J, et al. Comparison of three methods of targeting the subthalamic nucleus for chronic stimulation in Parkinson's disease. Neurosurgery. 2005;56(2 Suppl):360,8. discussion 360-8

24. Laxton AW, Tang-Wai DF, McAndrews MP, Zumsteg D, Wennberg R, Keren R, et al. A phase I trial of deep brain stimulation of memory circuits in Alzheimer's disease. Ann Neurol. 2010;68(4):521–34.
25. Gologorsky Y, Ben-Haim S, Moshier EL, Godbold J, Tagliati M, Weisz D, Alterman RL. Transgressing the ventricular wall during subthalamic deep brain stimulation surgery for Parkinson disease increases the risk of adverse neurological sequelae. Neurosurgery. 2011;69(2):294–9. discussion 299-300
26. Coenen VA, Gielen FL, Castro-Prado F, Abdel Rahman A, Honey CR. Noradrenergic modulation of subthalamic nucleus activity in human: metoprolol reduces spiking activity in microelectrode recordings during deep brain stimulation surgery for Parkinson's disease. Acta Neurochir. 2008;150(8):757,62. discussion 762
27. Konrad PE, Neimat JS, Yu H, Kao CC, Remple MS, D'Haese PF, et al. Customized, miniature rapid-prototype stereotactic frames for use in deep brain stimulator surgery: initial clinical methodology and experience from 263 patients from 2002 to 2008. Stereotact Funct Neurosurg. 2011;89(1):34–41.
28. Hutchison WD, Allan RJ, Opitz H, Levy R, Dostrovsky JO, Lang AE, et al. Neurophysiological identification of the subthalamic nucleus in surgery for Parkinson's disease. Ann Neurol. 1998;44(4):622–8.
29. Sterio D, Zonenshayn M, Mogilner AY, Rezai AR, Kiprovski K, Kelly PJ, et al. Neurophysiological refinement of subthalamic nucleus targeting. Neurosurgery. 2002;50(1):58–67; discussion 67-9.
30. Benazzouz A, Breit S, Koudsie A, Pollak P, Krack P, Benabid AL. Intraoperative microrecordings of the subthalamic nucleus in Parkinson's disease. Mov Disord. 2002;17(Suppl 3):S145–9.
31. Rodriguez-Oroz MC, Rodriguez M, Guridi J, Mewes K, Chockkman V, Vitek J, et al. The subthalamic nucleus in Parkinson's disease: somatotopic organization and physiological characteristics. Brain. 2001 Sep;124(Pt 9):1777–90.
32. Peppe A, Pierantozzi M, Bassi A, Altibrandi MG, Brusa L, Stefani A, et al. Stimulation of the subthalamic nucleus compared with the globus pallidus internus in patients with Parkinson disease. J Neurosurg. 2004 Aug;101(2):195–200.
33. Bejjani BP, Dormont D, Pidoux B, Yelnik J, Damier P, Arnulf I, et al. Bilateral subthalamic stimulation for Parkinson's disease by using three-dimensional stereotactic magnetic resonance imaging and electrophysiological guidance. J Neurosurg. 2000 Apr;92(4):615–25.

Subthalamic Nucleus DBS Placement for Parkinson's Disease: Use of the microTargeting™ Frame and Waypoint™ Stereotactic System with MER Guidance

3

Wendell Lake, Vishad Sukul, and Joseph S. Neimat

> **Core Messages**
> - The subthalamic nucleus (STN) target is frequently employed as a deep brain stimulation (DBS) target for the treatment of Parkinson's disease.
> - This target offers the advantage of tremor reduction and L-Dopa medication reduction.
> - When compared with other targets for the treatment of PD, such as the globus pallidus interna (GPi), some practitioners feel that the STN target may lead to greater reduction in impulse control, worsened cognitive deficits, and increased balance problems.
> - Modern rapid prototyping methods, such as 3D printing, have made it possible to create custom skull-mounted stereotactic mini-frames (microTargeting™ platform) specific to a given patient and target.
> - The microTargeting™ platform is a complete stereotactic system that offers several advantages including greater patient comfort, shorter surgical time on the day of lead implantation, reduced capital cost, and a shorter distance to target.
> - Disadvantages of the system include the requirement of an extra patient visit, because the frame must be planned with imaging on a day separate from the operative day, and some constraints on targeting trajectories on the day of surgery.

W. Lake
University of Wisconsin-Madison, Department of Neurosurgery, Madison, WI, USA

V. Sukul
Department of Neurosurgery, Albany Medical College, Albany, NY, USA

J. S. Neimat (✉)
Department of Neurological Surgery, University of Louisville, Louisville, KY, USA
e-mail: joseph.neimat@ulp.org

© Springer Nature Switzerland AG 2019
R. R. Goodman (ed.), *Surgery for Parkinson's Disease*,
https://doi.org/10.1007/978-3-319-23693-3_3

37

- Waypoint planning software is coupled with the microTargeting™ platform for the purpose of trajectory planning and frame creation.
- Waypoint planning software includes a probabilistic atlas based on a historical cohort of patients that previously underwent DBS placement, and it can be used as an adjunct to standardized coordinates in choosing the specific location of the STN target.
- After the trajectories are planned and the microTargeting™ frame is produced, it is affixed to the patients' skull on the day of lead placement. From this point, bur hole creation proceeds in the standard manner and microelectrode recording can occur simultaneously, if necessary, through both planned trajectories. Reducing the time necessary to affix the frame and plan the case on the day of surgery provides more time for MER and test stimulation and may improve patient cooperation, by shortening the surgical time.

Introduction

Currently, the STN is the structure most commonly targeted for DBS therapy of PD. The use of DBS therapy at the STN for PD first began in the early 1990s and was FDA approved in 2002. Although the exact mechanisms of DBS are incompletely understood, stimulation of the STN is thought to improve the symptoms of PD by blocking excessive output from the globus pallidus [1]. Some believe this may be accomplished by a temporary "lesioning" effect that interrupts the excitatory output of the STN to the GPi resulting in less thalamic inhibition and subsequently greater excitatory output to the cerebral cortex. However, much remains to be discovered regarding the mechanism of this therapy [2].

Stimulation of the STN has been shown to improve many of the symptoms of PD including tremor, bradykinesia, dyskinesia, and rigidity. Unfortunately, STN DBS may also be associated with side effects such as depressed mood, decreased visual processing speed, cognitive difficulty, and impulse control disorders. With appropriate patient selection and surgical technique, many of these side effects can be prevented and benefit can be maximized [3].

Traditional surgical technique for STN DBS lead placement generally involves application of a stereotactic frame to an awake patient followed by microelectrode recording (MER), test stimulation, final lead placement, and confirmatory testing of the position. Stereotactic guidance devices for DBS placement can be loosely categorized into two groups: frame-based and frame-less systems. Frame-based systems are the traditional devices which are affixed to the patient's head and the patient's head subsequently must be fixed in place to the OR table. Traditional stereotactic frames are generally relatively heavy metal fixtures that are affixed to the patient's head and scanned on the day of surgery with the frame and its fiducials in place, followed by frame adjustment to trajectory coordinates. Modern material science along with rapid prototyping techniques such as 3D printing now allows rapid production of disposable "frame-less" guidance systems. These smaller guidance devices are disposable, affix directly to the patients' skull, and because they are lighter do not require the patient to be rigidly locked to the OR table [4]. Two frameless systems commercially available are the Medtronic Nexframe™ and the FHC^R microTargeting™ frame (see FHC and Medtronic websites). These devices essentially co-opt the Cartesian coordinate space of volumetrically acquired CT or MRI scans and are smaller and lighter fixtures that improve patient comfort. One key difference between these two frameless options is the fact that the Nexframe requires active image guidance with a Stealth^R system, whereas the trajectories for the microTargeting™ platform are set at the time of its production and do not require image guidance during surgery [5]. While studies of the accuracy of frame-less systems and the traditional stereotactic frames demonstrate similar accuracy, we argue that the precision of the microTargeting™ system may be greater given the nature of its custom production providing a new frame each time and the fact that fewer user adjustments must be made since the trajectories are relatively set (as opposed to traditional frames which must be set each use and wear over time) [6]. This chapter will discuss the use of the microTargeting™ platform in conjunction with Waypoint™ stereotactic planning system for use in MER-guided STN DBS placement for the treatment of PD.

Operative Procedure for Use of the microTargeting™ Platform in STN DBS Lead Placement

The microTargeting™ platform used in conjunction with the Waypoint™ planning software is a complete stereotactic system. As such, it can be used for any number of stereotactic procedures with good accuracy and precision including placement of DBS leads or depth electrodes, tumor biopsy, or laser ablation [7]. In this chapter, we are specifically addressing the use of the microTargeting™ platform for placement of DBS leads at an STN target for the treatment of PD, but many of the principles are generalizable.

Patient Selection and Preoperative Concerns

Although discussed at length in other parts of this book, we will provide a brief comment on patient selection. Patient selection is an integral part of the surgical procedure. Patients with Parkinson's disease are typically considered DBS candidates when they develop significant on/off fluctuations in their symptoms despite a robust levodopa response, or have disabling dyskinesias. They must also have neuropsychological testing that precludes severe comorbid depression or progressive dementia and must be healthy enough to tolerate surgery without inordinate risk. In selecting the appropriate target for DBS, many centers now consider the STN and GPi to be similarly viable. Although practices differ, the STN may be preferred for patients with tremor predominance, high medication doses, or frequent wearing off. Patient factors such as major depression, cognitive difficulties, or excessive problems with gait may lead the team to consider a GPi target as opposed to STN [8]. In general, we have found that elderly patient's recover more slowly and are more prone to transient postoperative cognitive deficits. We commonly stage bilateral lead placement in patients over 70 years. The majority of our PD patients are treated with bilateral DBS unless their symptoms are predominantly one sided. DBS for PD should be a multidisciplinary process. The movement disorders neurologist, physical therapist/rehab team, and neuropsychologist are integral in the patient selection process, and decisions are typically made in a multidisciplinary conference.

Bone Marker Placement and Creation of the Frame

The first stage of STN DBS placement using the microTargeting™ platform is the placement of bone markers followed by imaging. The procedure can be performed under general or local anesthesia. The head is prepped and draped. Incision sites are infiltrated with local anesthetic. Four small stab incisions are created with an #10 scalpel blade, and one bone marker (5 mm Waypoint™ anchor) is placed at each site using an Osteomed screwdriver (Addison, TX, USA). Figure 3.1 demonstrates the appearance of bone markers on a typical CT with bone windows. Each incision site is closed with a skin staple. At our institution, a thin-cut noncontrasted CT scan of the head and a contrasted MRI of the brain is obtained, while the patient is under general anesthesia to limit artifact caused by tremor or involuntary patient movement. The CT scan is 512 × 512 pixels 0.5–1 mm slice thickness. The MRI is obtained on 1.5 or 3 T magnet and uses three-dimensional SPGR volumes, TR:

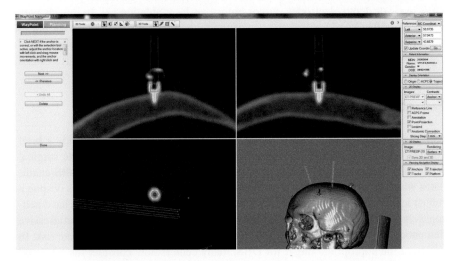

Fig. 3.1 microTargeting™ bone markers as viewed through the waypoint planning software

12.2, TE: 2.4; 256 × 256 × 170 voxels, and a voxel dimension of $1mm^3$. The patient is discharged the same day with oral pain medications as needed [4].

The imaging is loaded into a planning system for design of the frame. Although many commercially available systems are compatible with the microTargeting™ system, we use the Waypoint™ planning software that is available through FHC, Inc. (Bowdoin, Maine, USA). Once we have verified correct images and correct study date, we co-register the T1 with contrast and the T2 noncontrasted sequences to the thin-cut CT scan. The position of the bone markers is verified, and the positions of the AC, PC, and a midpoint (usually the falx) are selected. At this point, we select our target within the STN. At our center, the starting x, y, z coordinates of $(12,-3,-3)$ relative to the midcommisural point are used. Adjustments of the target are made by evaluating the position of the target within the STN as visualized on the T2 MRI sequences. Our center also uses probabilistic maps compiled from nonlinear imaging processing of the lead coordinates for a large cohort of patients who have previously undergone the STN DBS procedure [6]. A distillation of this information usually produces our final target position. With the target chosen, the entry point is selected in the region of the coronal suture. The specific trajectory chosen allows the electrode to reach its final target without injuring any vessels visible on the postcontrasted T1 MRI sequence (including cortical surface veins) and without violating the ependymal surface. Following the creation of trajectories, the Waypoint™ software generates a 3D model of the frame and it is checked to assure that frame is of appropriate configuration. Figure 3.2 provides a screenshot of trajectories in the Waypoint™ software and a frame model [4]. Once the frame is created in the planning software, the data can be transferred to the FHC server and the 3D frame can be generated, usually within 72 h. Prior to shipping, the frame is checked to assure accuracy. The frame should arrive 48 h prior to the lead placement

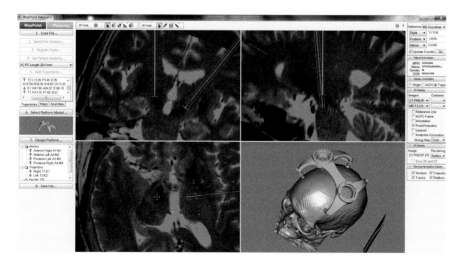

Fig. 3.2 Typical STN trajectories and a computer-generated frame model generated in waypoint planning software

to allow gas sterilization. Our workflow sequence usually involves placing the bone markers 1 week prior to lead placement. The frame plan is created the day following bone marker placement. The frame is generated and arrives at the OR facility 2–3 days prior to the lead placement. Since planning happens days before the operative procedure, we feel that it is easier to methodically plan the electrode trajectories without the time pressure and other distractions of a busy OR environment.

STN Lead Placement Using the microTargeting™ Platform

On the day of surgery, STN lead placement using the microTargeting™ platform is quite similar to the procedure as performed with a standard frame-based stereotactic system. Our standard procedure is to perform lead placement with the patient awake and off of any Parkinson's medication or medications that can affect tremor, including benzodiazepines. Dopaminergic medications are typically stopped the night before surgery.

At the time of the procedure, the patient is placed on the operating table supine in the beach chair position. The patient's head is prepped and draped. A clear plastic drape is applied and suspended above the patient's head so their vision is not obstructed. A short-acting IV opioid such as fentanyl is given at the beginning of the procedure to minimize discomfort while local anesthetic is injected. A mixture of lidocaine and bupivacaine is injected at each bone marker site. Epinephrine containing local anesthetic is used if the patients BP is well controlled, (<150 mmHg). The prior bone marker incisions are opened and step off screws are threaded into the bone marker screws. The frame is mounted after it is verified to be for the correct patient and the correct target. The scalp is marked at the appropriate point using a trocar touched to scalp and the exact point inked with a marking pen. Now the frame can be removed and the incisions created in a standard fashion. Now with the scalp opened the frame is re-mounted and the bone is marked with the trocar and a perforator is placed through the guidance tube portion of the frame and a standard bur hole is created in the frame trajectory. The dura is coagulated and opened. The surface of the brain is inspected, and any pial vessels underlying the bur hole are coagulated. Pia is opened in a cruciate fashion using an 11-blade scalpel.

The microdrive, set 10 mm above the target, is placed in a hub secured within the frame. We check with the anesthesiology team to assure that the patient's blood pressure is <140 mmHg and the microcanulla(s) are inserted. A mounted frame setup for MER is shown in Fig. 3.3 with only a single drive in place for illustrative purposes (in bilateral cases, we usually proceed with simultaneously mounted drives and MER). Microelectrode recording can proceed in a standard fashion from this point. We typically perform multitrack recording, often in the anterior, center, and posterior tracks of the rosette. Multitrack recording can quickly delineate the anatomy of the STN and may have the advantage of identifying relatively optimal tracks during comparative stimulation mapping. We seek a 4–6 mm span of STN with motor somatotopy and the typical increased firing rate seen in the STN. Driving down below the STN can provide further confirmation of position if substantia nigra recordings are obtained [4].

Fig. 3.3 The microTargeting™ platform mounted on a patient undergoing multitract MER with a single microdrive in place. Note that two microdrives can be mounted simultaneously for bilateral simultaneous MER

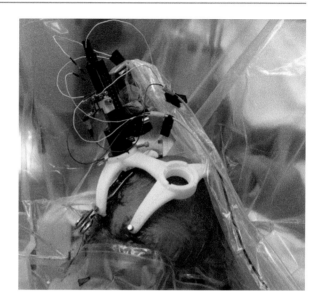

Following multitract MER, we perform further testing with semi-macro-stimulation after pulling back the MER leads. This stimulation testing allows evaluation of side effects such as eye deviation, muscle contraction, and others. Furthermore, test stimulation also allows some preliminary testing of efficacy. At each case, the intraoperative module of the Waypoint™ planning module is used to visualize the position of each tract. The software also allows one to enter MER data and test stimulation results relative to position [9].

Final lead position is determined based on a distillation of MER and test stimulation characteristics. With the final lead position chosen, we insert the final lead. For STN DBS cases, we typically use a Medtronic^R 3389 lead because the 7.5 mm span is sufficient for a small structure such as the STN. Once the final lead is positioned, we test each contact 0–3 using a monopolar from hundreds of implanted patients setting and slowly increasing the voltage. In doing this, we are predominantly testing for side effects. At that point, the lead is secured, typically in our cases with cement, but a securing cap can be used as well. The lead is carefully disengaged from the microdrive. The frame is removed, the leads positioned under the scalp appropriately, and the incisions closed. If a unilateral or bilateral case is done, the bone markers can be removed at this point. If a staged bilateral case is being done, the bone markers are left in place. The ability to reapply the frame without further adjustment in cases that are staged is a significant advantage of this system. The patient is generally brought back on a separate day for placement of the internal pulse generator and lead extensions.

Although the microTargeting™ platform does not offer the option of infinite trajectories, like a frame-based platform, standoff adjustments can achieve target adjustments of up to 11 mm in any direction. This has proven more than sufficient for the intraoperative adjustments that we have needed [4].

Advantages and Disadvantages of the microTargeting™ Stereotactic System

Our center has used the microTargeting™ stereotactic system extensively as have other high volume centers. This stereotactic system is increasing in popularity and is also used by centers that perform a lower volume of movement disorders surgery. Like all stereotactic systems, the microTargeting™ system has distinct advantages and disadvantages.

In general, all stereotactic systems must achieve a permissible level of accuracy, which is accepted to be in the submillimetric range. However, some may argue that the microTargeting™ system permits a higher level of precision, because each frame is custom created for the particular patient being treated. This removes the risk of human error during frame adjustments and the equipment is not subject to wear and need for maintenance [6]. Further precision advantages include a shorter distance to target, 120–130 mm compared to 180–190 mm for frame-based systems, such that small deviations are less consequential. No targeting scans are necessary the day of surgery so the amount of time the patient is awake in a frame and off medications is reduced by approximately 60–90 min. Reductions in operative time can increase patient comfort and minimize the strain on OR resources. Patient comfort may also be improved by the fact that the head is no longer rigidly fixed to the OR table. Since the patient is not fixed in a frame, access to the airway is unfettered and this improves safety. Finally, for lower volume centers, the capital cost necessary to use the microTargeting™ system is less than buying a frame-based system. This is important if relatively few movement disorder cases will be done but does represent a recurrent cost that must be weighed against gains in OR time for larger centers.

Disadvantages of the microTargeting™ platform are relatively few. Patients must make an additional trip to the center for placement of the bone markers and imaging on a week separate from the week of the procedure. For many patients, this is an acceptable trade-off for having a shorter awake procedure. Each bone marker placement requires a small stab incision, as opposed to the puncture site of the traditional frame-based systems. In general, these incisions can be placed behind the hairline and the cosmetic result is good. Finally, the OR materials team must have a system in place for verifying that the frame is received prior to the day of surgery for gas sterilization [4]. The cost of the frame, as noted above, may not compare favorably to the capital outlay for a traditional frame if the center is high volume.

Research Uses of the Waypoint™ Planning Software

For centers interested in research and quality analysis, the Waypoint™ planning software provides powerful data management capability. As previously mentioned, the intraoperative module of the Waypoint™ planner permits entering of MER and test stimulation data as well as virtual lead placement for overlay on the patients' anatomy. Data recorded within the planning software can be mined for research purposes and/or shared with other centers to create multicenter studies if desired.

Using active contact data from hundreds of implanted patients, at multiple centers, probabilistic maps, created by an image normalization algorithm, can be used to preoperatively plan DBS targets. At our center, standard STN coordinates, anatomical imaging, and probabilistic maps are used in conjunction to choose our lead target. With time, the research and data management capabilities associated with the Waypoint™ planning software continue to expand [10].

References

1. Benabid AL, Chabardes S, Mitrofanis J, Pollak P. Deep brain stimulation of the subthalamic nucleus for the treatment of Parkinson's disease. Lancet Neurol. 2009. https://doi.org/10.1016/S1474-4422(08)70291-6.
2. McIntyre CC, Savasta M, Kerkerian-Le Goff L, Vitek JL. Uncovering the mechanism(s) of action of deep brain stimulation: activation, inhibition, or both. Clin Neurophysiol. 2004. https://doi.org/10.1016/j.clinph.2003.12.024.
3. Charles D, Konrad PE, Neimat JS, et al. Subthalamic nucleus deep brain stimulation in early stage Parkinson's disease. Parkinsonism Relat Disord. 2012;20:731–7. https://doi.org/10.1016/j.parkreldis.2014.03.019.
4. Konrad PE, Neimat JS, Yu H, et al. Customized, miniature rapid-prototype stereotactic frames for use in deep brain stimulator surgery: initial clinical methodology and experience from 263 patients from 2002 to 2008. Stereotact Funct Neurosurg. 2011. https://doi.org/10.1159/000322276.
5. Kelman C, Ramakrishnan V, Davies A, Holloway K. Analysis of stereotactic accuracy of the cosman-robert-wells frame and nexframe frameless systems in deep brain stimulation surgery. Stereotact Funct Neurosurg. 2010;88(5):288–95. https://doi.org/10.1159/000316761.
6. D'haese PF, Pallavaram S, Konrad PE, Neimat J, Fitzpatrick JM, Dawant BM. Clinical accuracy of a customized stereotactic platform for deep brain stimulation after accounting for brain shift. Stereotact Funct Neurosurg. 2010. https://doi.org/10.1159/000271823.
7. Stuart RM, Goodman RR. Novel use of a custom stereotactic frame for placement of depth electrodes for epilepsy monitoring. Neurosurg Focus. 2008. https://doi.org/10.3171/FOC/2008/25/9/E20.
8. Follett KA, Weaver FM, Stern M, et al. Pallidal versus subthalamic deep-brain stimulation for Parkinson's disease. N Engl J Med. 2010;362:2077–91. https://doi.org/10.1056/NEJMoa0907083.
9. Camalier CR, Konrad PE, Gill CE, et al. Methods for surgical targeting of the stn in early-stage Parkinson's disease. Front Neurol. 2014. https://doi.org/10.3389/fneur.2014.00025.
10. Pallavaram S, D'Haese P-F, Lake W, Konrad PE, Dawant BM, Neimat JS. Fully automated targeting using nonrigid image registration matches accuracy and exceeds precision of best manual approaches to subthalamic deep brain stimulation targeting in Parkinson disease. Neurosurgery. 2015;1. https://doi.org/10.1227/NEU.0000000000000714.

Globus Pallidus Interna Deep Brain Stimulation: Practical Guide to Placement with Microelectrode Recording

4

Eric Hudgins, A. G. Ramayya, and G. H. Baltuch

> **Takeaways**
> - Both STN DBS and GPi DBS are approved by the Federal Drug Administration for use in PD.
> - The intended placement of the active DBS lead is in the motor territory of the GPi, approximately 3–4 mm from the border between the GPi and the internal capsule.
> - At our institution, we use the stereotactic frame-based approach to localize the GPi, both anatomically using MRI and physiologically using microelectrode recordings and stimulation.

Introduction

Surgical lesioning of the posterior globus pallidus interna (GPi), or pallidotomy, was performed in the 1950s to improve rigidity, tremor, and hypokinesia associated with Parkinson's disease (PD; [1, 6, 7, 11, 30]); however, this approach was abandoned after the introduction of Levadopa as an efficacious medical therapy in 1967 [5, 22]. Surgical treatment for PD re-emerged in the early 1990s as a result of several factors [13–15, 17, 18, 20, 21, 24, 25, 28, 29]. First, the limitations of medical therapy, such as failure to arrest disease progression, dyskinesias, and motor fluctuations, became apparent. Second, nonhuman primate studies demonstrated that parkinsonian motor symptoms were improved when lesions were applied to the GPi and the upstream subthalamic nucleus (STN), which were both pathologically hyperactive in the

E. Hudgins · A. G. Ramayya · G. H. Baltuch (✉)
Department of Neurosurgery, University of Pennsylvania, Philadelphia, PA, USA
e-mail: Gordon.Baltuch@uphs.upenn.edu

© Springer Nature Switzerland AG 2019
R. R. Goodman (ed.), *Surgery for Parkinson's Disease*,
https://doi.org/10.1007/978-3-319-23693-3_4

disease state ([2, 3, 8]). Third, advances in surgical technology such as stereotaxy, intraoperative electrophysiology, and magnetic resonance imaging (MRI) allowed for the creation of safe, reversible, and titratable effects via deep structures using chronic high-frequency deep brain stimulation (DBS; [4, 5, 9, 10]). STN DBS was first reported in a PD patient by Benabid in 1993 [23] and GPi DBS was first reported by Siegfried and Lippitz in 1994 [26]. Several randomized clinical studies have demonstrated that STN DBS and GPi DBS are more effective than medical therapy alone and are both approved by the Federal Drug Administration for use in PD (see [22], for a review). This chapter will detail our method for the effective targeting of GPi by using Leksell frame stereotactic coordinates and microelectrode recording for placement of DBS leads (or macroelectrodes). A more detailed description of the general technique of DBS implantation at our institution has been previously described [16].

Stereotactic Targeting of the GPi

The intended placement of the active DBS lead is in the motor territory of the GPi, approximately 3–4 mm from the border between the GPi and the internal capsule. Various localization approaches can be used to target the GPi, including frame-based approaches, frameless neuronavigation-guided approaches using a skull-mounted frame, rather than a traditional stereotactic frame, and using real-time guidance with intraoperative MRI [31]. At our institution, we use a frame-based approach with the *Leksell Micro Stereotactic System Model G Frame* (Elekta) for stereotactic targeting of the GPi. The polar coordinate system of the Leksell frame provides an effective strategy for reaching deep brain targets, while also avoiding superficial cortical vessels [19, 27]. The frame is positioned to be precisely midline, using the lateral canthi and zygomatic arches as landmarks [16]. After applying the frame, two MRI sequences are obtained using a 1.5-T magnet (Signa, General Electric), a 1.3-mm slice T1-weighted MRI scan with gadolinium contrast to aid in *indirect* targeting, and a 2.5 mm T2-weighted MRI scan to aid in *direct* targeting, both described below. The frame coordinate system is established by manually identifying the frame's localizer markings on an MRI scan that is co-registered to a brain atlas (see [16] for details). For reference, the X coordinate marks mediolateral, the Y coordinate marks anterioposterior, and the Z coordinate marks the superioinferior dimension, respectively. X, Y, Z of 0, 0, 0 represents the right-most, posterior-most, and superior-most point on the frame and 100,100,100 marks the center of the frame. A manual correction is made so that 100,100,100 corresponds with the midcommissural point, or the midpoint of a line drawn between the anterior commissure (AC) and the posterior commissure (PC, AC-PC line). If there is a large discrepancy between the center of the frame and the midcommissural point, the frame must be repositioned with new screw sites. We anatomically localize the GPi using a combination of *direct* and *indirect* targeting, which involves using MRI to identify an X, Y, Z coordinate for the GPi within the frame coordinates. *Indirect* targeting involves identifying the GPi relative to the midcommissural point (17–21 mm lateral, 2 mm anterior, and 5 mm inferior) on a T1-weighted MRI, whereas the *direct* targeting method involves identifying the GPi on an axial slice of a T2-weighted MRI scan, about 5 mm below the AC-PC line, that allows for anatomical localization of subcortical structures.

Setting the Electrode Trajectory

Once the target site for the DBS lead has been identified, an electrode trajectory or angle of approach is determined. The trajectory to the target site consists of the *azimuth,* or the angle of approach in the mediolateral plane, and the *declination*, or the angle of approach in the anterior-posterior plane. We use the StimPilot system (Medtronic, Inc.) to plan the trajectory. The StimPilot system uses the MRI scan of the patient with the frame placed in its current position. The polar coordinate system of the Leksell frame is reestablished by manually marking the frame's localizer positions on the MRI scan. The AC, PC, and target site are remeasured using indirect and direct techniques described above. Briefly, the indirect method involves identifying the GPi relative to the midpoint of the AC-PC line identified on T1-weighted MRI (using predefined coordinates), whereas the direct method involves identifying the GPi using direct anatomical identification on a T2-weighted scan. In practice, the target is initially calculated by the indirect technique and then may be adjusted, based on the identification of the GPi on the T2 axial images (the direct approach). Next a trajectory is set so as to avoid the lateral ventricles if possible and to avoid any veins on the cortical surface (best visualized using a T1-weighted MRI scan with contrast). Finally, lateral C-arm fluoroscopy is used to ensure that the lead makes a direct path to the target and for verification of target depth, as the electrode is advanced into the brain (Fig. 4.1).

Fig. 4.1 Lateral radiograph through Leksell frame showing macroelectrode in target position at center

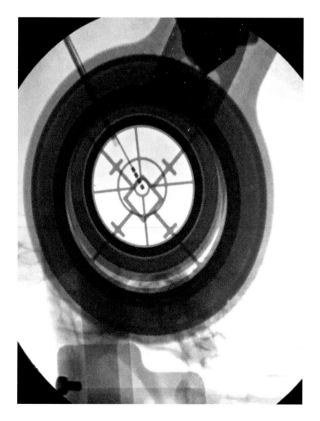

Microelectrode Recording and Stimulation to Physiologically Target the GPi

Following target planning using direct and indirect methods as described above, microelectrode recordings along the planned electrode trajectory can verify the targeting of the posteroventral GPi. Microelectrode recordings allow for localization with a high spatial resolution and can account for factors that may result in inaccurate targeting, such as brain shift. We use a microdrive system (FHC positioner, Frederick Haer, Bowdoinham, ME) that is mounted on the stereotactic frame and incorporates a Ben-Gun guide that allows for insertion of a guide tube via one or more holes for microelectrode tracts (a central hole and holes that are 2 mm anterior, posterior, lateral, and medial to the center). A 1-μm tungsten microelectrode is introduced through the central hole; the ground electrode attaches to the guide cannula whereas the recording electrode attaches to the distal tip of the microelectrode. Before advancing the microelectrode, it is important to ensure that the microelectrode guide tube does not abut the dural edges, as even a minimal force can deviate the tube and compromise targeting. To eliminate unnecessary forms of electromagnetic interference, all lights, suction devices, electronic operating table, and Bovie electrocautery are turned off. The microelectrode is advanced to target depth and confirmed with C-arm fluoroscopy at 10, 5, and 2 mm above the target depth, to ensure an appropriate trajectory. The nonsterile physiology team assists the surgical team by performing sensorimotor tests at various points along the electrode trajectory.

While driving the microelectrode into the GPi and recording extracellular single and multiunit action potentials, one will encounter several physiological patterns [31]. First, one should encounter striatum (caudate or putamen), which mostly consists of neurons with low spontaneous discharge rates (0–10 Hz). Next, one will encounter GPe neurons that have spontaneous discharge rates of 30–60 Hz and typically fire in a "bursting" or "pausing" pattern in PD patients. GPi neurons, in contrast, demonstrate high tonic firing rates from 60–100 Hz. Border cells are typically located between the GPe and GPi and can provide a distinct clue that the microelectrode will soon enter the GPi. Border cells have a 10–20 Hz firing pattern and a high signal-to-noise ratio (Fig. 4.2). Within the posteroventrolateral GPi, sensorimotor activity may be identified by passive and active movement of the contralateral joints increasing unit discharges [12]. While driving the microelectrode and recording activity, positioning a flashing light above the patient's eyes allows the neurophysiologist and surgeon to detect visual-evoked activity (time-synced to the flashing light) prior to reaching the optic tract and minimize the chance of entering the optic tract and helps avoid ventral misplacement. The optic tract is typically about 1.5 mm below the ventral border of the GPi [12].

Microstimulation can be used to confirm appropriate placement in the GPi. Correct placement of the microelectrode in the GPi will result in improvement in cogwheel rigidity with stimulation. Inappropriate placement ventrally into the optic tract can produce flashing-light phenomena (phosphenes) in the contralateral visual hemifield. Placement medial to the ideal target will position the electrode within the

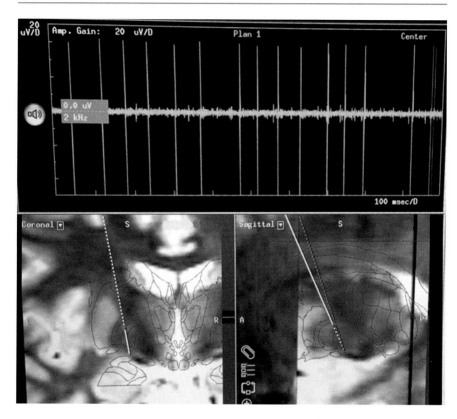

Fig. 4.2 Electrophysiologic characteristics of GPi, demonstrating correct localization using microelectrode. MRI co-registered with a Sterotactic atlas demonstrates the electrode tip to be located within GPi (red dot) on the coronal image

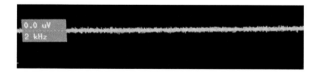

Fig. 4.3 Low signal-to-noise ratio consistent with medial placement of the microelectrode within the posterior limb of the internal capsule

posterior limb of the internal capsule, in which case microelectrode electrophysiology will show a low signal-to-noise ratio consistent with white-matter recording (Fig. 4.3). Stimulation at low currents (e.g., 10 μA at 300 Hz, 200 μs pulse width) will then produce contralateral muscle contractions [31]. Anterior, dorsal, lateral misplacement will position the electrode within the external segment of the globus pallidus (GPe), which in most cases produces no effect on the patient during stimulation. In some situations, however, there might be an improvement in PD motor symptoms.

Once the target coordinates are confirmed anatomically and physiologically, the microelectrode is removed from the guide cannula and a quadripolar DBS lead (Medtronic, Inc.) is advanced along the same track to the desired electrode depth. C-arm fluoroscopy is used to confirm an appropriate trajectory and depth. Finally, macrostimulation through the DBS lead is used to confirm appropriate placement, by assessing for improvement in symptoms and for adverse effects. Details regarding closure, bilateral placement, and placement of the implantable pulse generator (IPG) have been described previously [16].

Conclusion

In our experience, targeting GPi employing direct and indirect stereotactic guidance, microelectrode recording, and micro- and macrostimulation provides a safe and accurate means for placement of deep brain stimulation electrodes. Microelectrode recordings display characteristic signals of the target structure, the GPi, as well as nearby structures. The preferred therapeutic target for placement of the macroelectrode is within the posteroventrolateral GPi, where sensorimotor activity is often present. Morphological differences between patients can make targeting this area challenging. However, the combined use of MRI Leksell frame stereotactic anatomic guidance and microelectrode recording and stimulation, to optimize GPi targeting, can overcome this challenge.

References

1. Alkhani A, Lozano AM. Pallidotomy for parkinson disease: a review of contemporary literature. J Neurosurg. 2001;94(1):43–9.
2. Bergman H, Wichmann T, DeLong MR. Reversal of experimental parkinsonism by lesions of the subthalamic nucleus. Science. 1990;249(4975):1436–8.
3. Benazzouz A, Gross C, Feger J, Boraud T, Bioulac B. Reversal of rigidity and improvement in motor performance by subthalamic high-frequency stimulation in MPTP-treated monkeys. Eur J Neurosci. 1993;5:382–9.
4. Benabid AL, Pollak P, Louveau A, Henry S, de Rougemont J. Combined (thalamotomy and stimulation) stereotactic sur- gery of the VIM thalamic nucleus for bilateral Parkinson disease. Appl Neurophysiol. 1987;50(1–6):344–6.
5. Benabid AL. Deep brain stimulation for Parkinson's disease. Curr Opin Neurobiol. 2003;13(6):696–706.
6. Blomstedt P, Hariz GM, Hariz MI. Pallidotomy versus pallidal stimulation. Parkinsonism Relat Disord. 2006;12(5):296–301.
7. Bronstein JM, DeSalles A, DeLong MR. Stereotactic pallidotomy in the treatment of Parkinson disease: an expert opinion. Arch Neurol. 1999;56(9):1064–9.
8. DeLong MR. Primate models of movement disorders of basal ganglia origin. Trends Neurosci. 1990;13(7):281–5.
9. Gironell A, et al. Effects of pallidotomy and bilateral subthalamic stimulation on cognitive function in Parkinson disease: a controlled comparative study. J Neurol. 2003;250(8): 917–23.

10. Gironell A, et al. Motor circuitry re-organization after pallidotomy in Parkinson disease: a neurophysiological study of the bereitschaftspotential, contingent negative variation, and N30. J Clin Neurophysiol. 2002;19(6):553–61.
11. Guridi J, Lozano AM. A brief history of pallidotomy. Neurosurgery. 1997;41(5):1169–83.
12. Gross RE, et al. Electrophysiological mapping for the implantation of deep brain stimulators for Parkinson's disease and tremor. Mov Disord. 2006;21(14):259–83.
13. Hariz MI, Bergenheim AT. A 10-year follow-up review of patients who underwent Leksell's posteroventral pallidotomy for Parkinson disease. J Neurosurg. 2001;94(4):552–8.
14. Jacques DS, Eagle KS, Kopyov OV. Use of posteroventral pallidotomy for treatment of Parkinson's disease: is pallidotomy still an experimental procedure? A review and commentary. Stereotact Funct Neurosurg. 1998;70(1):19–31.
15. Kleiner-Fisman G, et al. Long-term effect of unilateral pallidotomy on levodopa-induced dyskinesia. Mov Disord. 2010;25(10):1496–8.
16. Kramer DR, Halpern CH, Buonacore DL, McGill KR, Hurtig HI, Jaggi JL, Baltuch GH. Best surgical practices: a stepwise approach to the University of Pennsylvania deep brain stimulation protocol. Neurosurg Focus. 2010;29(2):E3.
17. Krauss JK, et al. Posteroventral medial pallidotomy in levodopa-unresponsive parkinsonism. Arch Neurol. 1997;54(8):1026–9.
18. Laitinen LV, Bergenheim AT, Hariz MI. Ventroposterolateral pallidotomy can abolish all parkinsonian symptoms. Stereotact Funct Neurosurg. 1992;58:14–21.
19. Leksell L, et al. A new fixation device for the Leksell stereotaxic system. Technical note. J Neurosurg. 1987;66(4):626–9.
20. Lozano AM, Lang AE. Pallidotomy for Parkinson's disease. Neurosurg Clin N Am. 1998;9(2):325–36.
21. Melnick ME, et al. Effect of pallidotomy on postural control and motor function in Parkinson disease. Arch Neurol. 1999;56(11):1361–5. Available at: http://www.ncbi.nlm.nih.gov/pubmed/10555656.
22. Miocinovic S, Somayajula S, Chitnis S, Vitek JL. History, applications, and mechanisms of deep brain stimulation. JAMA Neurol. 2013;70(2):163–71.
23. Pollak P, Benabid AL, Gross C, et al. Effets de la stimulation du noyau sous thalamique dans la maladie de Parkinson. Rev Neurol (Paris). 1993;149(3):175–6.
24. Quinn N. Progress in functional neurosurgery for Parkinson's disease. Lancet. 1999;354(9191):1658–9.
25. Siegel KL, Metman LV. Effects of bilateral posteroventral pallidotomy on gait of subjects with Parkinson disease. Arch Neurol. 2000;57(2):198–204.
26. Siegfried J, Lippitz B. Bilateral chronic electrostimulation of ventroposterolateral pallidum: a new therapeutic approach for alleviating all parkinsonian symptoms. Neurosurgery. 1994;35:1126–9.
27. Simon SL, et al. Error analysis of MRI and Leksell stereotactic frame target localization in deep brain stimulation surgery. Stereotact Funct Neurosurg. 2005;83(1):1–5.
28. Sobstyl M, et al. Bilateral pallidotomy for the treatment of advanced Parkinson disease. Neurol Neurochir Pol. 2003;37(Suppl 5):251–62.
29. Soukup VM, et al. Cognitive sequelae of unilateral posteroventral pallidotomy. Arch Neurol. 1997;54(8):947–50.
30. Spiegel EA, Wycis HT, Szekely EG, et al. Stimulation of Forel's field during stereotaxic operations in the human brain. Electroencephalogr Clin Neurophysiol. 1964;16:537–48.
31. Starr PA. Pallidal interventions for Parkinson's disease. In: Winn HR, editor. Youmanns neurological surgery. 6th ed. New York: Elsevier; 2011. p. 938–43.

Microelectrode Recording-Based Targeting for Parkinson's Disease Surgery

5

Charles B. Mikell III and Joseph S. Neimat

Core Messages
- Microelectrode recording (MER) is a key technique for electrode targeting in deep brain stimulation surgery.
- MER depends on an experienced practitioner differentiating signature forming patterns of basal ganglia structures.
- The targets in Parkinson's disease are the subthalamic nucleus (STN), the globus pallidus internus (GPi), and, rarely, the ventral intermediate nucleus of the thalamus (VIM) or the posterior subthalamic area (PSA), which includes the caudal zona incerta.
- The keys to identification of dorsal STN are neuronal firing rate, firing pattern, and passive motion sensitivity.
- The keys to identification of GPi are identification of globus pallidus externus and the optic tract.
- The value of MER has been questioned and is evolving.

Introduction

Microelectrode recording (MER) has a long history in neurosurgery and has paralleled the development of stereotactic targeting of subcortical structures. MER is a critical step in mapping subcortical structures. It is accomplished by comparing the

C. B. Mikell III
Department of Neurosurgery, Stony Brook University Hospital, Stony Brook, NY, USA

J. S. Neimat (✉)
Department of Neurological Surgery, University of Louisville, Louisville, KY, USA
e-mail: joseph.neimat@ulp.org

© Springer Nature Switzerland AG 2019
R. R. Goodman (ed.), *Surgery for Parkinson's Disease*,
https://doi.org/10.1007/978-3-319-23693-3_5

Fig. 5.1 A typical trajectory to subthalamic nucleus. Care is taken to enter a gyrus rather than a sulcus. We typically begin mapping 10–15 mm above target. The thalamus can be seen adjacent to the third ventricle. (Figure is from Camalier et al. 2014)

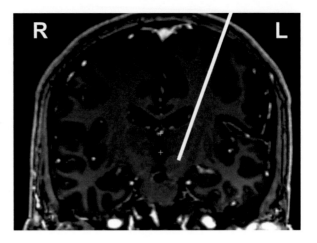

basal firing rates and response properties of detected structures to the known regional anatomy. Done correctly, MER thus provides a detailed understanding of both the anatomy and physiological function of circuits relevant to movement disorders. For instance, the identification of tremor cells in the subthalamic nucleus (STN) both suggests that the identified location is likely to be an effective location for permanent placement of the deep brain stimulation (DBS) electrode and hints at the pathophysiology of tremor in Parkinson's disease (PD) [1]. Despite advances in intraoperative neuroimaging that have called its use into question [2], MER's ability to physiologically verify DBS targets continues to have broad application among functional neurosurgeons (Figs. 5.1 and 5.2).

In this chapter we will briefly explore the history of MER before describing the technical basics of MER, as practiced in 2018. We will discuss the relevant subcortical anatomy of the STN and the globus pallidus internus (GPi), the most frequent surgical targets in PD, as well as discuss some less frequently used targets. We will close with a discussion of novel techniques in MER, including automated target detection and closed-loop systems.

History

Spiegel and Wycis developed frame-based stereotaxy for the treatment of psychiatric disease and reported this advance in *Science*, in 1947 [3, 4]. However, they quickly realized that individual anatomy was variable and looked for techniques to improve the precision of targeting [5]. Albe-Fessard was the first to use MER to map the human thalamus [6], but her papers were mostly published in French, and her findings did not reach a wide, English-speaking audience. However, in the 1980s, DeLong and colleagues applied these techniques to primate basal ganglia physiology [7] and used insights gained in this manner to develop a detailed map of the functional organization of the human STN and pallidum [8]. These techniques were then applied by Kelly and others to create reproducible lesions of the thalamus

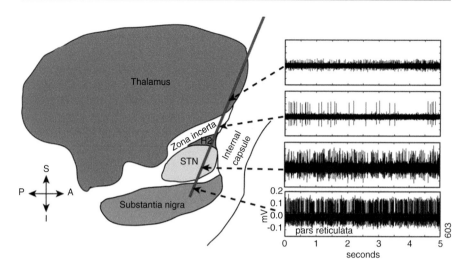

Fig. 5.2 Multiunit activity in subcortical structures has distinct firing rates and patterns. In the thalamus, firing rates of 15–25 Hz, including both bursting and nonbursting cells, are typical. There is rarely neuronal activity in the zona incerta. STN is identifiable by its marked increase in background and firing rates from 35–45 Hz. Finally, the substantia nigra contains tonically active cells firing at variously reported rates from 30–70 Hz. (Figure is from Camalier et al. 2014)

[9] and pallidum [10]. Roughly contemporaneously, Alim Benabid in Grenoble observed that high-frequency stimulation could have clinical benefits similar to lesion generation in both PD and ET [11]. Alim Benabid's group eventually used MER to guide DBS surgery of the thalamus [12], as well as STN surgery [13]. Indeed it was the use of intraoperative stimulation used for mapping that led to the observation that high-frequency stimulation could "create a functional lesion" and led to the advent of DBS. At present, MER is widely used in these surgeries.

Advantages of MER

Stereotactic targeting is a messy business, as there remains significant disagreement on how and where to target standard BG structures. Indirect methods with averaged coordinates as well as "direct" targeting of MRI-identifiable structures are available [14]. MER provides the ability to directly identify neuronal populations with defined characteristics, including firing rate and bursting behavior. Moreover, somatotopic features of STN, ventralis intermedius (VIM) nucleus, and other targets can be used to confirm that the targeted region subserves parts of the body that are afflicted by bothersome symptoms, like tremor or dyskinesia. For instance, in the treatment of hand tremor by VIM stimulation, it is believed that the best treatment efficacy results from stimulating parts of VIM that respond to passive hand or wrist movements [15]. Although this confirmatory function can be somewhat replicated without MER by placing the permanent electrode and stimulating it, or performing macrostimulation of the cannula, there is appeal to using the smaller MER electrodes before passing the larger cannula or test electrode. As above, there is no class I evidence to confirm this suspicion.

A second advantage of MER is that a second practitioner may be engaged in the surgery. Many successful DBS programs include a neurologist who performs the intraoperative neurophysiology, as well as grades the response to test stimulation intraoperatively. In our experience, two heads are better than one in DBS, and a second experienced physician or neurophysiologist can often confirm clinical suspicions or detect subtle abnormalities that the operating surgeon would fail to detect during the procedure. This collaborative approach with the movement disorders neurologist can provide more comprehensive consideration of the patient's symptoms and is appreciated by the patient. Often this practitioner is interested in MER from a research perspective, as well.

A third advantage of MER (which accrues to society) is the research that has been conducted on neural structures targeted in DBS. Our understanding of how cortical-basal ganglia loops contribute to behavior in normal and pathological states has been greatly expanded by insights from DBS surgery. More recently, studies interrogating the anterior cingulate gyrus [16] and the prefrontal cortex [17] in behaving patients have been possible. While individual patients rarely directly benefit from the MER research in which they participate, new therapies are being developed using signals identified in DBS. This would not have been possible without MER.

Disadvantages of MER

Obvious downsides of MER are (1) the additional time required, (2) the additional passes through the brain with the microelectrodes, and (3) the cost of the equipment, neurophysiology personnel, and OR time needed for mapping. However, whether these issues are themselves associated with risk remains unsettled. To be sure, time of the operation has been associated with infection in one large series [18], but this has not been uniformly reproduced [19]. It is not clear, additionally, that image-guided surgeries are significantly faster; in one recent report of asleep, CT-guided surgery, operative time was somewhat longer than the time needed for more traditional, MER-guided surgery (190 versus 145 min [20]. Yet it is certain that long procedures are taxing for the patient as well as the practitioner. Whether long duration is itself associated with medical risk is not clear.

The risk associated with multiple penetrations through the brain seems self-evident, but the actual numbers are not clear. In one report, multiple penetrations were associated with hemorrhage risk [2], a finding that has been reproduced in some [21] (in one case not at the 0.05 p value level) [22] but not all reports [23, 24]. Some of the discrepancies may be due to differences in cannula size used by some centers employing MER (i.e., smaller MER cannulas may not engender the same risk as the larger DBS lead cannula). Eskandar and colleagues reported improvement in hemorrhage rates when the electrodes were redesigned, so that only the microwire tip is advanced through the brain rather than the microelectrode along with its protective sleeve. However, a recent systematic review did conclude that MER increased hemorrhage risk [25] and concluded that image-guided techniques are therefore preferred. This claim is highly controversial, given the long history of MER use and the lack of strong evidence that imaging-based targeting is superior [26]. Nonetheless, it is beyond dispute that MER is associated with some risk of hemorrhage.

MER Basics

MER depends upon identifying and recording subtle changes in membrane potential that are characteristic of action potentials and postsynaptic potentials in local neuron populations (including the typical DBS targets). This is typically done with thin, tungsten-coated electrodes attached to a differential amplifier, which is accompanied by various bells and whistles, depending on the manufacturer. These signals are typically unique to different brain regions, and trained neurophysiologists interpret these signals as "fingerprints" of subcortical structures, including the STN, GPi, thalamus, and so on. After a structure is identified, its response properties can also be determined, including its response to active or passive joint movements, sensory input, flashing lights, and so on. Taken together, the neurosurgeon can use this information to assemble a detailed picture of the anatomy and physiology of the interrogated region.

Neurophysiological Signals Relevant to DBS

The signal most commonly used to guide mapping for DBS surgery is high-frequency activity (>300 Hz) corresponding to multiunit activity (MUA). MUA corresponds to the action potential firing of a local group of neurons, and its frequency and pattern are characteristic of the STN, thalamus, substantia nigra, and other subcortical structures. A variety of tricks are used to amplify it over the rest of the broadband signal, especially hardware high-pass filtering. The signal amplitude itself is quite modest (as one would expect from individual neurons!), and is easily drowned out by electrical or mechanical noise, if care is not taken in the recordings. Nonetheless, with care, attention, and the right equipment, it is straightforward to detect and characterize MUA.

A second signal that is robustly identified is referred to as the background. The background appears to represent synaptic activity and distant action potential firing that is still identifiable despite the use of filtering and high-impedance electrodes that only detect a small area. A marked, sudden increase in amplitude of the background characterizes the STN [27], and attempts have been made to detect this phenomenon in an automated way [28].

Hardware Needed

Modern neurophysiology equipment consists of four parts: recording electrodes (typically made of tungsten), a headstage containing a preamplifier (and sometimes a hardware high-pass filter), an analog-to-digital conversion board, and a computer where the digital signals are turned into sound and visual representations for interpretation by a neurophysiologist. Commercial systems to do this include the Neuro Omega™ by Alpha Omega (Nazareth, Israel) and the Guideline 4000 LP+™ by FHC (Bangor, ME). These systems are essentially similar in capability and pricing.

Personnel Needed

In addition to a neurosurgeon, a trained neurophysiologist is typically needed to interpret the MUA and background signals to construct a detailed, three-dimensional map of recorded structures. There is no accepted, standard training for DBS neurophysiologists; they may be engineers, PhD neuroscientists, or physicians (neurosurgeons or neurologists typically with experience in a basic neurophysiology research laboratory). However, only a physician may bill insurers a professional fee, in accordance with federal guidelines, and the fee for MER interpretation cannot be billed by the neurosurgeon who is billing for the surgery. Other professionals may collect reimbursement out of the hospital's diagnosis-related group fee. The neurophysiologist will typically have a detailed understanding of the regional anatomy being interrogated. He or she will also have experience in the technical aspects of neurophysiology, especially in understanding how to improve the signal-to-noise ratio. Finally, this team member must be comfortable in the operating room, sometimes for lengthy periods, while mapping is underway.

Targets in PD

Typical targets for the treatment of PD include STN, GPi, and, occasionally, VIM thalamus, as well as investigational targets including the posterior subthalamic area (PSA), which includes the caudal zona incerta, and the pedunculopontine nucleus (PPN).

STN MER

Basic Procedure for Identifying STN   The surgeon will generally create a stereotactic plan, which is implemented using frame-based or frameless stereotaxy. A tract is planned that typically passes through striatum, thalamus, zona incerta (ZI), STN, and substantia nigra. Using the surgeon's preferred technique, a burr hole aligned with the planned trajectory is created, and a cannula is passed to some fixed distance (typically 25, 15, or 10 mm) above target. Longer trajectories take longer to map, but may provide more detailed anatomical information. The microelectrode(s) (from one to five electrodes) is/are then passed downward to and through the target. After identification of STN (or whatever structures happen to be identified), a decision is made about whether to pass the microelectrode(s) along an additional track or tracks or to place the stimulating electrode in the identified target. If the decision is made to attempt a different trajectory, the cannula or cannulas will be reintroduced, usually 2 mm away from the prior track(s), and the process is repeated. Many centers incorporate macrostimulation (of the guide sleeve) or microstimulation (of the tungsten microelectrode) into this paradigm.

Neurophysiology of the Ideal Tract In the ideal pass, the striatum, thalamus, ZI, STN, and substantia nigra are all encountered at the expected depths.

Before Encountering STN In a typical tract, started 10–20 mm above target, the neurosurgeon will encounter the lateral part of the thalamus. Its neurophysiology is characterized by two cell types, bursting and nonbursting cells, at a density of approximately two cells per millimeter, and an overall mean firing rate between 15 and 25 Hz [29]. More specifically, the bursting cells are reported to have a mean firing rate of ~15 Hz, and the nonbursting cells fire at ~28 Hz [30]. These are reported to correspond to the reticular, ventralis oralis anterior, or lateropolaris nuclei. Background activity is relatively low. The ZI is encountered next. The ZI is a thin rim of gray matter between the thalamus and subthalamus which may treat tremor when stimulated [31, 32]. However, it is identifiable by its paucity of neuronal activity.

STN After the ZI is traversed, there is typically a massive increase in action potential firing and background activity. This marks the superior boundary of the STN. Sources vary about the mean firing rate, reported between 35 and 45 Hz, but agree that a variety of regular and irregularly firing neurons are present [27, 29, 30]. Recordings are continued until there is a decrease in background activity, corresponding to exit from the STN [29]. Subsequent to this, the substantia nigra pars reticulata (SNpr) is identified. SNpr is distinctive because of its tonic pattern of discharge variously reported between 30 and 70 Hz [27, 30] and has been compared to the sound of rain on a tin roof (Okun M, Personal communication). SNpr lacks kinesthetic responses and is not typically mapped in detail.

STN has extensive kinesthetic responses, especially rostrally and dorsally. This anteromedial location is believed to be the most effective location for stimulation therapy and corresponds to the sensorimotor territory of the STN [33]. In general, STN cells respond to movement of contralateral limbs across one or two joints, and responses tend to be relatively clear. The proportion of STN cells reported with kinesthetic responses varies between 26 % and 40 % in the literature [27, 30]. These responses are absent from SNpr, which also indicates exit from STN.

Stimulation Testing While it is good to identify efficacy with intraoperative testing, a variety of issues prevent full assessment of clinical efficacy in the operating room, including patient comfort and the use of sedation. In a responsive patient, however, significant improvements in rigidity or tremor are good signs of an effective placement. It is important to note however that while immediate effects may be a good predictor, they are not invariably identical to the effects of long-term stimulation.

If side effects are detected at low stimulation amplitude, the electrode should be moved. The STN is bordered anteriorly and laterally by motor fibers from the internal capsule, medially by fibers in CN III, and posteriorly by the medial lemniscus. Therefore, face pulling or dysarthria should prompt posterior or medial movement. Eye movement abnormalities indicate too medial a trajectory. Contralateral paresthesia should prompt movement forward. If some clinical benefit is identified, and there are no side effects, the electrode should be fixed into place.

Debugging a Suboptimal STN Recording Suboptimal recordings are either (1) technically bad or (2) fail to detect adequate STN. From a technical standpoint, the most common issue is line noise, from any of numerous sources in the operating room, especially the cauteries and the electric drill. These should be unplugged. Loud, repetitive noises known as "ground loops" are a consequence of high-amplitude signals oscillating in the amplifier. Ensuring adequate grounding prevents this issue. Other technical issues should be discussed with the MER equipment manufacturer.

When not enough (or no) STN is detected, Bakay has developed an algorithm, depending on the other MER findings, and microstimulation [33]. If microstimulation triggers the above events, the appropriate maneuvers should be made. If microstimulation is not available, or has no acute effect, the length of time spent in the thalamus should be considered, as well as the distance between the thalamus and STN. If the thalamic pass is long, one is either medial or posterior, as distinguished by the distance between the thalamus and STN. If this distance is long, one is posterior, and if it is short, medial. Alternately, if the thalamic pass is short, one is either anterior or lateral, possibilities which are again distinguished by distance between the STN and thalamus (long distance is consistent with an anterior tract, and short is probably lateral). If no STN is encountered, one is either anterior or posterior, possibilities again distinguished by how much thalamus was recorded.

GPi MER

For a variety of reasons, including mood disorders and cognitive disorders, a GPi target may be considered in some patients [34]. MER for GPi is straightforward but does have some technical nuance. Most passes begin in the striatum, which exhibits tonic firing at 4–6 Hz. Subsequent to this, the globus pallidus externus (GPe) is entered. GPe is characterized by two types of units: high-frequency bursting neurons, separated by pauses (60 Hz), or lower-frequency neurons (10–20 Hz) with periods of bursting [35, 36]. There is typically a 1–2 mm area characterized by decreased activity or border cells (firing regularly at 20–40 Hz) corresponding to the medial medullary lamina that is encountered before the GPi is encountered [35]. GPi neurons have a firing rate (80–90 Hz) a bit higher than GPe, which is qualitatively similar to STN [35, 37], with high cellular density. The sensorimotor territory of GPi is found posteroventrally. Approximately 25% of neurons in this area have kinesthetic responses, which should be looked for [35]. Below the inferior border of GPi is the optic tract. Visual evoked responses are often seen in this location and should be considered confirmatory of a good pass. The final target should have the first contact of the DBS electrode just over the optic tract, with the other contacts in the posteroventral GPi.

Debugging a Suboptimal GPi Recording Technical issues should be addressed as above. We adapt another algorithm from Bakay, if little or limited kinesthetically responsive GPi neurons are identified. GPi is bounded anteriorly and laterally by GPe and posteriorly and medially by the corticospinal tract. If microstimulation elicits contralateral movements, the length of the GPi pass should be considered. If GPi itself was short, one is probably posterior and should move 2 mm anterior. If no movements are elicited by microstimulation, the width of the medial medullary lamina should be considered. If it was long (4–6 mm), one is probably too lateral and should move 2 mm medially. Otherwise, it is likely one is anterior and should move posteriorly. Anterior tracts may detect basal forebrain cells that have a high tonic firing rate and no kinesthetic responses.

Other Targets in PD

VIM nucleus of the thalamus is the oldest target for PD tremor, and it is still a reasonable choice for tremor-dominant disease [12]. Many centers place VIM electrodes without MER, but if MER is desired, the essential step is to identify sensory thalamus (Vc thalamus) and place the electrode 2–3 millimeters anterior [33]. PPN is an investigational target for treatment of freezing and gait disturbance in PD. It consists of populations of cholinergic and glutamatergic neurons, which are responsible for gait initiation and voluntary movement initiation, respectively [38]. PPN is located medial and inferior to SNpr and is usually approached almost directly from a lateral angle. Its units have a firing rate around 15 Hz and some subtle kinesthetic responses [39]. PPN surgery is best performed under an institutional review board protocol, under the guidance of physicians from an experienced center. The posterior subthalamic area is a location that includes caudal zona incerta, and has been stimulated in tremor syndromes that are not traditionally responsive to VIM stimulation, including postural tremors that occasionally accompany PD [40].

Future Directions in MER

In the setting of advancing neuroimaging technology, there are strong incentives to prove the usefulness of MER in the operating room. Several recent developments have demonstrated potential new directions for MER in stereotactic surgery. One promising technique is performing MER under light general anesthesia. The efficacy of this technique may be comparable to awake surgery [41]. Along these lines, there is experience using automated techniques to detect boundaries of the STN, which may take the human error out of neurophysiology [42]. Finally, use of field potentials, rather than MUA, has permitted the development of closed-loop systems that stimulate in response to brain activity rather than in a continuous fashion [43]. The coming years will no doubt bring further advances of this kind.

References

1. Levy R, Hutchison WD, Lozano AM, Dostrovsky JO. High-frequency synchronization of neuronal activity in the subthalamic nucleus of parkinsonian patients with limb tremor. J Neurosci. 2000;20(20):7766–75. PubMed PMID: 11027240.
2. Burchiel KJ, McCartney S, Lee A, Raslan AM. Accuracy of deep brain stimulation electrode placement using intraoperative computed tomography without microelectrode recording. J Neurosurg. 2013;119(2):301–6. https://doi.org/10.3171/2013.4.JNS122324. PubMed PMID: 23724986.
3. Gildenberg PL. Spiegel and Wycis—the early years. Stereotact Funct Neurosurg. 2001;77(1–4):11–6. PubMed PMID: 12378049.
4. Spiegel EA, Wycis HT, Marks M, Lee AJ. Stereotaxic apparatus for operations on the human brain. Science. 1947;106(2754):349–50. PubMed PMID: 17777432.
5. Spiegel EA. Methodological problems in stereoencephalotomy. Confin Neurol. 1965;26(3):125–32. PubMed PMID: 5329807.
6. Albe-Fessard D, Arfel G, Guiot G, Derome P, Guilbaud G. Thalamic unit activity in man. Electroencephalogr Clin Neurophysiol. 1967;Suppl 25:132+. PubMed PMID: 4165777.
7. DeLong MR, Crutcher MD, Georgopoulos AP. Primate globus pallidus and subthalamic nucleus: functional organization. J Neurophysiol. 1985;53(2):530–43. PubMed PMID: 3981228.
8. Lenz FA, Vitek JL, DeLong MR. Role of the thalamus in parkinsonian tremor: evidence from studies in patients and primate models. Stereotact Funct Neurosurg. 1993;60(1–3):94–103. Review. PubMed PMID: 8511438.
9. Kelly PJ, Ahlskog JE, Goerss SJ, Daube JR, Duffy JR, Kall BA. Computer-assisted stereotactic ventralis lateralis thalamotomy with microelectrode recording control in patients with Parkinson's disease. Mayo Clin Proc. 1987;62(8):655–64. PubMed PMID: 2439850.
10. Lozano AM, Lang AE, Galvez-Jimenez N, Miyasaki J, Duff J, Hutchinson WD, Dostrovsky JO. Effect of GPi pallidotomy on motor function in Parkinson's disease. Lancet. 1995;346(8987):1383–7. PubMed PMID: 7475819.
11. Benabid AL, Pollak P, Louveau A, Henry S, de Rougemont J. Combined (thalamotomy and stimulation) stereotactic surgery of the VIM thalamic nucleus for bilateral Parkinson disease. Appl Neurophysiol. 1987;50(1–6):344–6. PMID: 3329873.
12. Benabid AL, Pollak P, Gervason C, Hoffmann D, Gao DM, Hommel M, Perret JE, de Rougemont J. Long-term suppression of tremor by chronic stimulation of the ventral intermediate thalamic nucleus. Lancet. 1991;337(8738):403–6. PubMed PMID: 1671433.
13. Limousin P, Krack P, Pollak P, Benazzouz A, Ardouin C, Hoffmann D, Benabid AL. Electrical stimulation of the subthalamic nucleus in advanced Parkinson's disease. N Engl J Med. 1998;339(16):1105–11. PubMed PMID: 9770557.
14. Andrade-Souza YM, Schwalb JM, Hamani C, Eltahawy H, Hoque T, Saint-Cyr J, Lozano AM. Comparison of three methods of targeting the subthalamic nucleus for chronic stimulation in Parkinson's disease. Neurosurgery. 2008;62(Suppl 2):875–83. PubMed PMID: 15794832.

15. Lozano AM, Hutchison WD, Dostrovsky JO. Microelectrode monitoring of cortical and sub-cortical structures during stereotactic surgery. In: Meyerson BA, Ostertag C, editors. Advances in stereotactic and functional neurosurgery 11. New York: Springer Vienna; 1995. p. 30–4.
16. Sheth SA, Mian MK, Patel SR, Asaad WF, Williams ZM, Dougherty DD, Bush G, Eskandar EN. Human dorsal anterior cingulate cortex neurons mediate ongoing behavioural adaptation. Nature. 2012;488(7410):218–21. https://doi.org/10.1038/nature11239. PubMed PMID: 22722841.
17. Mian MK, Sheth SA, Patel SR, Spiliopoulos K, Eskandar EN, Williams ZM. Encoding of rules by neurons in the human dorsolateral prefrontal cortex. Cereb Cortex. 2014;24(3):807–16. https://doi.org/10.1093/cercor/bhs361. PubMed PMID: 23172774.
18. Tolleson C, Stroh J, Ehrenfeld J, Neimat J, Konrad P, Phibbs F. The factors involved in deep brain stimulation infection: a large case series. Stereotact Funct Neurosurg. 2014;92(4):227–33. https://doi.org/10.1159/000362934. Review. PubMed PMID: 25096381.
19. Sillay KA, Larson PS, Starr PA. Deep brain stimulator hardware-related infections: incidence and management in a large series. Neurosurgery. 2008;62(2):360–7. https://doi.org/10.1227/01.neu.0000316002.03765.33. PubMed PMID:18382313.
20. Gorgulho A, De Salles AA, Frighetto L, Behnke E. Incidence of hemorrhage associated with electrophysiological studies performed using macroelectrodes and microelectrodes in functional neurosurgery. J Neurosurg. 2005;102(5):888–96. PubMed PMID: 15926715.
21. Xiaowu H, Xiufeng J, Xiaoping Z, Bin H, Laixing W, Yiqun C, Jinchuan L, Aiguo J, Jianmin L. Risks of intracranial hemorrhage in patients with Parkinson's disease receiving deep brain stimulation and ablation. Parkinsonism Relat Disord. 2010;16(2):96–100. https://doi.org/10.1016/j.parkreldis.2009.07.013. PubMed PMID: 19682943.
22. Deep-Brain Stimulation for Parkinson's Disease Study Group, Obeso JA, Olanow CW, Rodriguez-Oroz MC, Krack P, Kumar R, Lang AE. Deep-brain stimulation of the subthalamic nucleus or the pars interna of the globus pallidus in Parkinson's disease. N Engl J Med. 2001;345(13):956–63. PubMed PMID: 11575287.
23. Binder DK, Rau GM, Starr PA. Risk factors for hemorrhage during microelectrode-guided deep brain stimulator implantation for movement disorders. Neurosurgery. 2005;56(4):722–32. PubMed PMID: 15792511.
24. Ben-Haim S, Asaad WF, Gale JT, Eskandar EN. Risk factors for hemorrhage during microelectrode-guided deep brain stimulation and the introduction of an improved microelectrode design. Neurosurgery. 2009;64(4):754–63. https://doi.org/10.1227/01.NEU.0000339173.77240.34. PubMed PMID: 19349834.
25. Zrinzo L, Foltynie T, Limousin P, Hariz MI. Reducing hemorrhagic complications in functional neurosurgery: a large case series and systematic literature review. J Neurosurg. 2012;116(1):84–94. https://doi.org/10.3171/2011.8.JNS101407. Review. PubMed PMID: 21905798.
26. Montgomery EB Jr. Microelectrode targeting of the subthalamic nucleus for deep brain stimulation surgery. Mov Disord. 2012;27(11):1387–91. https://doi.org/10.1002/mds.25000. PubMed PMID: 22508394.
27. Benazzouz A, Breit S, Koudsie A, Pollak P, Krack P, Benabid AL. Intraoperative microrecordings of the subthalamic nucleus in Parkinson's disease. Mov Disord. 2002;17(Suppl 3):S145–9. PubMed PMID: 11948769.
28. Snellings A, Sagher O, Anderson DJ, Aldridge JW. Identification of the subthalamic nucleus in deep brain stimulation surgery with a novel wavelet-derived measure of neural background activity. J Neurosurg. 2009;111(4):767–74. https://doi.org/10.3171/2008.11.JNS08392. PubMed PMID: 19344225.
29. Sterio D, Zonenshayn M, Mogilner AY, Rezai AR, Kiprovski K, Kelly PJ, Beric A. Neurophysiological refinement of subthalamic nucleus targeting. Neurosurgery. 2002;50(1):58–69. PubMed PMID: 11844235.
30. Hutchison WD, Allan RJ, Opitz H, Levy R, Dostrovsky JO, Lang AE, Lozano AM. Neurophysiological identification of the subthalamic nucleus in surgery for Parkinson's disease. Ann Neurol. 1998;44(4):622–8. PubMed PMID: 9778260.

31. Plaha P, Khan S, Gill SS. Bilateral stimulation of the caudal zona incerta nucleus for tremor control. J Neurol Neurosurg Psychiatry. 2008;79(5):504–13. PubMed PMID: 18037630.
32. Fytagoridis A, Sandvik U, Aström M, Bergenheim T, Blomstedt P. Long term follow-up of deep brain stimulation of the caudal zona incerta for essential tremor. J Neurol Neurosurg Psychiatry. 2012;83(3):258–62. https://doi.org/10.1136/jnnp-2011-300765. PubMed PMID: 22205676.
33. Bakay RA, editor. Movement disorder surgery: the essentials. New York: Thieme; 2009.
34. Follett KA, Torres-Russotto D. Deep brain stimulation of globus pallidus interna, subthalamic nucleus, and pedunculopontine nucleus for Parkinson's disease: which target? Parkinsonism Relat Disord. 2012;18(Suppl 1):S165–7. https://doi.org/10.1016/S1353-8020(11)70051-7. Review. PubMed PMID: 22166422.
35. Lozano AM, Hutchison WD. Microelectrode recordings in the pallidum. Mov Disord. 2002;17(Suppl 3):S150–4. PubMed PMID: 11948770.
36. Guridi J, Gorospe A, Ramos E, Linazasoro G, Rodriguez MC, Obeso JA. Stereotactic targeting of the globus pallidus internus in Parkinson's disease: imaging versus electrophysiological mapping. Neurosurgery. 1999;45(2):278–89. PubMed PMID: 10449072.
37. Hutchison WD, Lozano AM, Davis KD, Saint-Cyr JA, Lang AE, Dostrovsky JO. Differential neuronal activity in segments of globus pallidus in Parkinson's disease patients. Neuroreport. 1994;5(12):1533–7. PubMed PMID: 7948856.
38. Pahapill PA, Lozano AM. The pedunculopontine nucleus and Parkinson's disease. Brain. 2000;123(Pt 9):1767–83. Review. PubMed PMID: 10960043.
39. Mazzone P, Lozano A, Stanzione P, Galati S, Scarnati E, Peppe A, Stefani A. Implantation of human pedunculopontine nucleus: a safe and clinically relevant target in Parkinson's disease. Neuroreport. 2005;16(17):1877–81. PubMed PMID: 16272871
40. Plaha P, Ben-Shlomo Y, Patel NK, Gill SS. Stimulation of the caudal zona incerta is superior to stimulation of the subthalamic nucleus in improving contralateral parkinsonism. Brain. 2006;129(7):1732–47.
41. Fluchere F, Witjas T, Eusebio A, Bruder N, Giorgi R, Leveque M, Peragut JC, Azulay JP, Regis J. Controlled general anaesthesia for subthalamic nucleus stimulation in Parkinson's disease. J Neurol Neurosurg Psychiatry. 2014;85(10):1167–73. https://doi.org/10.1136/jnnp-2013-305323. PubMed PMID: 24249783.
42. Wong S, Baltuch GH, Jaggi JL, Danish SF. Functional localization and visualization of the subthalamic nucleus from microelectrode recordings acquired during DBS surgery with unsupervised machine learning. J Neural Eng. 2009;6(2):026006. https://doi.org/10.1088/1741-2560/6/2/026006. PubMed PMID: 19287077.
43. Rosin B, Slovik M, Mitelman R, Rivlin-Etzion M, Haber SN, Israel Z, Vaadia E, Bergman H. Closed-loop deep brain stimulation is superior in ameliorating parkinsonism. Neuron. 2011;72(2):370–84. https://doi.org/10.1016/j.neuron.2011.08.023. PubMed PMID: 22017994.

MRI-Guided DBS for Parkinson's Disease

6

Richard Rammo, Jason M. Schwalb, and Ellen L. Air

Key Points
- Accurate implantation of deep brain stimulation leads can be performed using real-time MRI guidance while the patient is under general anesthesia.
- Patient selection and target choice follow standard paradigms.
- MRI safety is of primary importance in the planning and execution of the procedure.
- Outcomes of iMRI-guided placement are equivalent to traditional approaches.

Introduction

Successful treatment of Parkinson's disease (PD) by deep brain stimulation (DBS) relies on stimulation of a physiologically responsive location within the brain, which in turn requires accurate DBS electrode/lead placement. For the two targets most commonly used for the treatment of PD, the subthalamic nucleus (STN) and globus pallidus interna (GPi), experience has taught us the most effective region for stimulation within each structure [21, 6, 18]. Reaching these targets requires a means to relate an external apparatus (typically, a stereotactic frame secured to the skull) with the deep internal structures of the brain. The stereotactic frame, in

R. Rammo · E. L. Air (✉)
Department of Neurosurgery, Henry Ford Hospital, Detroit, MI, USA
e-mail: eair1@hfhs.org

J. M. Schwalb
Department of Neurosurgery, Henry Ford West Bloomfield Hospital,
West Bloomfield, MI, USA

© Springer Nature Switzerland AG 2019
R. R. Goodman (ed.), *Surgery for Parkinson's Disease*,
https://doi.org/10.1007/978-3-319-23693-3_6

combination with imaging, has allowed surgeons to precisely implant electrodes/ leads and perform other stereotactic procedures with adequate accuracy and relative ease [5].

Despite its ability to reach a given target with pinpoint (1–2 mm, in general) accuracy, the frame does have its disadvantages. First, securing the frame onto an awake patient is uncomfortable and can be stressful for patients, particularly those with claustrophobia or anxiety. Second, the pre-operative target localization does not account for intra-operative brain shift that occurs with CSF egress and air ingress. The degree to which this happens in a particular patient cannot be predicted [9, 11, 12]. The resultant shift typically is of the anterior commissure (AC) posteriorly, in the direction of gravity, with little change in the posterior commissure (PC), leading to shortening of the AC–PC distance. This can lead to suboptimal targeting and poor clinical outcomes [9, 12]. Medial–lateral shifting can also occur. Third, errors in manipulation or setting of the frame can produce targeting inaccuracy. To correct for the possible brain shift and mechanical errors, many surgeons employ micro-electrode recording (MER) to refine the target based on neuronal activity [1, 3, 8, 18], though there remains controversy concerning its necessity [10]. The success of the frame-based MER approach typically requires an awake, cooperative patient who has been without dopaminergic medication on the day of the surgery. Most patients tolerate this approach, with coaching and reassurance, while some require deep sedation and in some cases the procedure must be aborted. Some patients avoid surgery altogether due to fear of undergoing an awake brain surgery. Therefore, the ability to account for brain shift and confirm lead placement using direct intra-operative visualization provides an alternative approach for successful DBS implantation [14, 16].

Patient Selection

As with any approach to DBS, the success of the intra-operative MRI (iMRI)-guided procedure begins with appropriate patient selection. Our approach is similar to that detailed in Chap. 1, with a multi-disciplinary team of specialists assessing each patient for motor response to levodopa, absence of "red flags" that indicate an alternative diagnosis, and lack of significant cognitive dysfunction. Appropriate patient expectations are established. It is confirmed that the individual's goals for treatment are aligned with anticipated clinical benefits. It should be emphasized that DBS is a long-term commitment that requires ongoing treatment to achieve the best outcome.

In our experience, the prospect of an asleep approach to DBS has led patients who were previously unwilling to consider surgery to seek surgical consultation. We have also worked with many anxious patients who, with education, have become willing participants in an awake procedure. We welcome those for whom the iMRI approach brought them to discuss DBS, but advise them regarding both iMRI and frame-based placement. Because the procedure is performed under general anesthesia and patients may take their dopaminergic medications the morning of surgery, we have found the iMRI approach particularly suited for patients with claustrophobia, significant anxiety, or severe pain/discomfort in their "off" state. In the absence of a contraindication to iMRI, patient preference also guides this choice.

Contraindications to the iMRI approach are related to MRI safety and risks of general anesthesia. As with MRI-guided frame-based surgery, a complete MRI safety check must be completed to determine the compatibility of any implanted devices and implants (e.g., automatic internal cardiac defibrillator or spinal cord stimulator) and exclude retained metal (e.g., shrapnel). The specifics of your iMRI magnet and head coil must be cross-checked with implanted devices to determine if compatible. Keep in mind that most "MRI compatible" implants are currently rated against a 1.5 T magnet strength and a send–receive head coil [17].

The most recent generation of DBS hardware offers improved MRI compatibility. Therefore, staged implantation, with implantation of the IPG between cranial procedures, can now be offered. Compatibility between the specific make and model of implanted hardware and the iMRI system being used must be confirmed before proceeding with the implantation of additional electrodes using this approach.

The risk of general anesthesia must also be considered when determining the best approach for DBS implantation. Patients with mild pulmonary or cardiac disease may have lower risk of morbidity with an awake surgical approach. Medical conditions which place a patient at significant surgical risk, such as poorly controlled diabetes, significant pulmonary or cardiac disease, and history of non-healing wounds, are relative contraindications for DBS placement, independent of the surgical approach.

MRI System Requirements

MRI-guided DBS implantation can be successfully performed in either a diagnostic scanner or one that is part of an operative suite, as long as the core requirements are met. This includes the ability to ensure a sterile field, to accommodate required anesthesia equipment, and the installation of a waveguide that allows connection between MRI safe and unsafe portions of operative equipment (e.g., bipolar electrocautery). Furthermore, an MRI-compatible drill and titanium instruments are necessary (i.e., forceps, scissors, rongeurs, etc.) [24]. Your institution's MRI safety officer should be involved in purchase decisions and guide the team in maintaining an MRI-safe environment.

Currently, the only commercial system available for iMRI DBS implantation is the ClearPoint® System produced by MRI Interventions, Inc. It has been successfully used in both 1.5 T and 3 T MRI units, and is compatible with all available MRI manufacturers. The system hardware includes a laptop computer with ClearPoint® software, MRI compatible monitor and control pad that allow navigation of the software from within the MRI room, and adjustable head fixation frame. The ClearPoint® software supports all aspects of the procedure from surgical planning to target navigation and confirmation of final lead placement. The surgical kit includes the required disposables, which will be further discussed below.

Pre-operative Preparation

As there are many important details, we have found the use of a checklist extremely helpful in ensuring a smooth and successful procedure. The case begins with appropriate set-up of the MRI suite. Because most MRI scanners are used for both diagnostic imaging and surgical procedures, care must be taken to establish a clean operative environment, by wiping down all surfaces, before surgical equipment is brought into the suite. We recommend placing clear adhesive plastic drapes and/or towels around the integrated frame and coil, to reduce soiling. A final safety check of all instruments and equipment is performed before they are brought into the MRI suite. Instruments should be kept in separate surgical trays and each individual instrument clearly marked as MRI-safe. Titanium instruments are typically identifiable as having a different color from standard instruments, however, additional marking is encouraged.

Patients are advised to take their Parkinson's medications as typically scheduled on the day of surgery. Once the patient is under general anesthesia, clippers are used to remove hair. A wide strip spanning the coronal suture is required, though many prefer to clip the entire scalp. Then we infiltrate the wide strip of the scalp with local anesthetic. Performing this step prior to bringing the patient into the scanner aids hemostasis as MRI-safe bipolar forceps tend not to be as efficient as those used in a standard operating room. It is important to not forget at this time to place earplugs in the patient's ears. Next, the patient's head can be secured in the integrated head frame (Fig. 6.1a). The ideal position is slightly extended and offset to the left. This best accommodates the skull-mounts and typically avoids collision between the frame and the MRI bore. The top of the patient's head should be positioned in the rostral–caudal direction at the center of the head coil. This optimizes visualization of both intracranial structures and the mounted frame. Finally, anesthesia should be able to access the patient at all times, although this may be a challenge, depending on the length of the bore. A final check of the patient is performed to ensure monitoring cords are without loops and are padded from the patient, to prevent heat conduction and burning during the procedure.

Procedure

Draping and Initial Trajectory Planning

The patient is brought into the MRI bore, with the head initially brought to the operative end of the bore. The surgical site is prepped in the usual fashion. A special drape with accordion feature is placed, which maintains sterility at the operative end of the magnet and of the patient's head as it moves within the bore [24]. Elastic bands on the drape secure it to each end of the bore. Once the patient is draped, MRI visible marking grids are placed over the anticipated burr hole site(s), typically centered just in front of the coronal suture (Fig. 6.2a). The patient is then returned to bore-center.

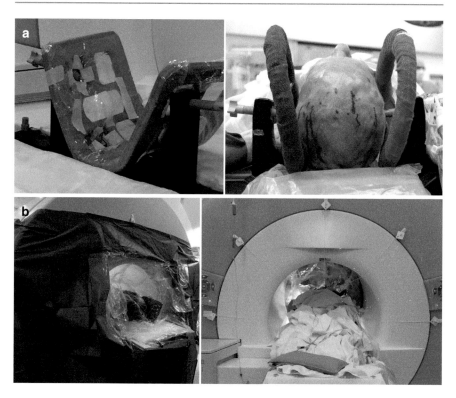

Fig. 6.1 Positioning and Draping: Head fixation frame is secured to the table and MRI coil placed within it (**a**, left). Head is positioned within the frame and coils (**a**, right). Two different styles of flexible head coils are shown and will vary by MRI system. The accordion drape is placed after prepping, covering the working area at the head (**b**, left), with elastic bands secured to the foot end of the bore to allow movement of the drape with movement of the patient (**b**, right)

A T1-weighted, post-contrast, volumetric scan (T1W) is performed and transferred into the ClearPoint® software. The software will present auto-detected anterior commissure (AC) and posterior commissure (PC) locations, which are easily adjusted as needed by the user. A mid-sagittal point must also be defined, best placed near bregma. Initial target(s) and trajectory planning is then performed. As standard targets (STN and GPi) are not well-defined on T1W images, indirect targeting relative to the AC–PC plane is entered into the system at this stage. Further sequences which better visualize the target will be obtained in later steps that allow for fine-tuning of the exact target.

Alternatively, the ClearPoint® software allows for pre-operative scans to be imported and targeting performed on the appropriate sequences. The AC–PC coordinates of the defined targets are saved in the software, then transferred onto the T1W images obtained at surgery. We routinely obtain a volumetric MRI as part of our pre-operative patient evaluation, so it is readily available for import. Pre-planning the target in advance saves time during the trajectory planning step. Focus can then be turned to optimizing the trajectory. One can toggle between probe and

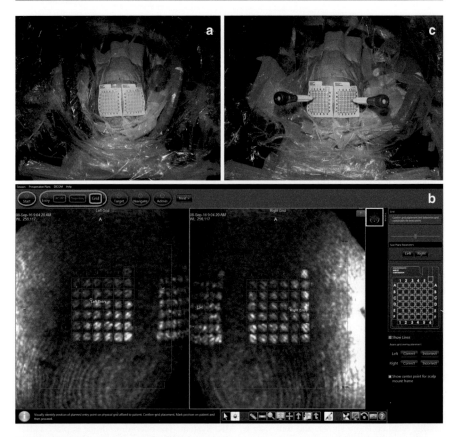

Fig. 6.2 Marking the Opening: MRI visible grids are placed over the anticipated entry point on each side (**a**), which are then detected by the Clearpoint® software (**b**). The entry point is indicated by the software. Once the top portion of the grid is removed, the marking tools can be placed through the skin and into the bone at the specified location (**c**)

anatomical views to best visualize the relationship of the trajectory to sulci, ventricles, and vessels. After confirming the trajectory, the software will present the optimal location to center the incision, burr hole, and frame relative to the MR-visible scalp grid (Fig. 6.2b).

Opening and Frame Placement

The top layer of the scalp grid is removed, leaving the white portion on the scalp. A marking tool is then placed through the indicated point on the grid, through the skin, and into the bone. The marking tool should be advanced until it is firmly seated in the bone (tool will stay in position without being held, Fig. 6.2c). This ensures that a distinct hole will be made in the bone beneath. The marking tool and grid are then removed, and skin incision made. A linear or curvilinear incision can be made

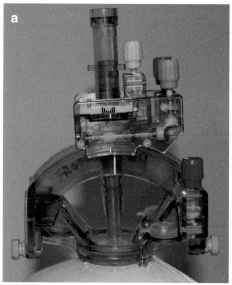 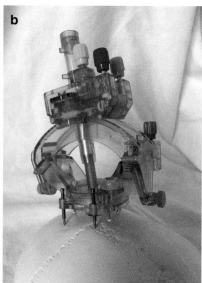

Fig. 6.3 Types of Smartframe® bases: The skull-base mounted frame (**a**) sits directly on the skull and requires 5–6 cm incision. The scalp-base mounted frame (**b**) is secured to the skull through the skin, offset to account for its higher pivot point. A smaller incision can be used, tailored to the procedure

depending upon the surgeon's preference. Some variations in frame placement, incision, and workflow exist depending on the type of ClearPoint Smartframe® used (Fig. 6.3).

The basic components of the Smartframe® system are the base, either scalp or skull mounted, and the arc. The skull-mounted frame must be seated directly onto the skull, requiring an approximate 5 cm incision. The scalp-mounted frame is secured to the skull through the skin, requiring a much smaller incision. The frame base is positioned relative to the bone divot made by the marking tool and secured with the pre-loaded screws. Check to make sure the frame base does not rock. The MRI fiducials on the base should be checked to ensure fluid is present in each. Although interchangeable, we prefer to mount the base first, then drill the burr hole.

When creating the burr hole, it is essential to undercut the inner table to avoid bone collision, particularly along the planned trajectory. The Stimloc® base is placed over the burr hole, the dura and pia are opened and coagulated. The Smartframe® arc is then placed onto the frame and secured. Check that the X–Y stage is set to 0–0 (yellow and green lines aligned in the center) and the alignment stem is in down position with fluid in stem. Place but do not tighten locking screw. The hand controller is then connected to the arc, aligning each color-coded end.

The patient is moved to isocenter and a T1 volumetric scan is performed with additional slices to include the frame base and alignment stem. Then, appropriate sequences are performed to highlight the target (T2 or inversion recovery), which are fused to the volumetric scan. Based on these images obtained after frame placement and dural opening, final targeting is performed. Scan parameters for these and all the procedural scans can be found in [24] and in the iBook by Larson, Starr, and Martin [15], though optimized parameters have also been developed for each MRI system by MRI Interventions.

Alignment

Once final targeting is completed, the software will provide scan plane parameters that must be entered into your MRI system. These direct 2D imaging slabs identify the location of the alignment stem relative to the frame base and predict the size and direction of error (Fig. 6.4). The system then calculates and directs adjustments to be made using the hand controller. The arc allows for four directions of adjustment: pitch, roll, X, and Y. Pitch and roll are used to make larger adjustments in the A–P and medial–lateral directions, respectively. The X–Y stage allows for fine adjustments. Due to the limited range of the X–Y stage (2.5 mm in each direction), pitch and roll should be used to align the system to less than 1.0 mm predicted error from the target. The sequences obtained during the X–Y adjustment step are more accurate than those for the pitch and roll step. Therefore the predicted error on an X–Y scan may be larger than 1.0 mm, despite a smaller predicted error at the prior step. In this case, the system can provide additional pitch and roll adjustments until the error is small enough to move to X–Y adjustments. A locking screw should be secured prior to moving to the X–Y adjustment step.

Of note, the entry point remains that defined at the initial trajectory step. However, on occasion, it is necessary to adjust the entry point due to the final seating of the base and small shifts at the cortical surface. This can be accomplished by adjusting the X–Y stage. The software will aid in compensating for such adjustment through subsequent steps.

The cycle of short MRI alignment scans and manual adjustments is continued until the radial error is sufficiently small, generally less than 0.4 mm. Experience with your institutions' system, and from those with similar scanners elsewhere, may reveal the system to have a directional bias in final lead location, e.g., final lead location is consistently 0.2 mm posterior to that predicted prior to insertion. Such biases should be considered when determining the amount and direction of error you are willing to accept before moving to the insertion step.

Insertion

When you have determined you are ready to place the lead, the software will provide the insertion length to be marked with a depth-stop on the blunt-tipped ceramic stylet. The stylet is then placed into the peel-away sheath and its holder, and the

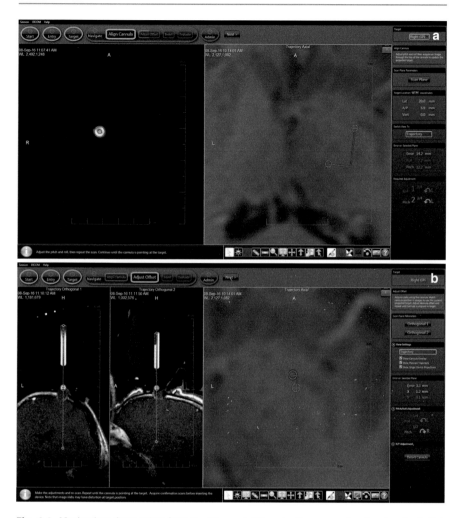

Fig. 6.4 Navigation: Screenshot from the Clearpoint® navigation computer showing the initial images performed after frame placement (**a**). The alignment stem is detected (left) and the required adjustments calculated (right). The cross-hair indicates the intended target, while the open circle indicates the detected trajectory of the alignment stem. Following pitch and roll adjustments, orthogonal slab images are obtained which provide increased accuracy (**b**). The current location of the alignment stem is again detected (left) and the required adjustments indicated (right). These can be made using either pitch and roll or the X–Y stage as illustrated (right)

sheath is adjusted until the tip of the stylet is exposed (Fig. 6.5). The stylet is then advanced into the brain. If the pia has been sufficiently opened, the stylet should pass smoothly. A sharp-tipped stylet is included, and may be used to ensure the pia is opened at the entry point. If the stylet still does not pass smoothly, the entry point must be inspected for collision with the bone edge. Some prefer to use the sharp stylet to open the dura and pia at the time of lead placement, rather than open these at the beginning of the case. However, the success of this approach requires the

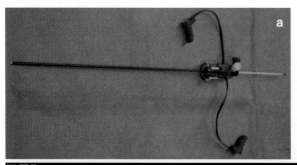

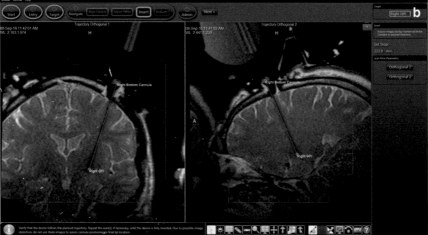

Fig. 6.5 Insertion: The peel-away sheath is assembled with the ceramic stylet inserted (**a**). The tip of the ceramic stylet should just protrude from the bottom of the sheath. Once inserted, the stylet can be visualized on slab images to confirm it followed the correct trajectory (as indicated by the yellow line, Fig. 6.5b)

opening to be precisely along the intended trajectory, without deviation caused by bowing of the stylet while attempting to pass through a tough dura. Deviation at the point of entry has been the single greatest cause of lead misplacement, so attention to the bony, dural, and pial openings is critical. We standardly obtain a short scan after partial insertion of the stylet to confirm that no deviation has occurred, before advancing the stylet to target.

At target, a confirmation scan is obtained which reveals the radial error at the target, as well as the depth. This scan is most helpful in calculating the depth to be measured on the electrode, so the desired contact is placed at the targeted depth. When keen attention has been paid to the details of the preceding steps, we have not had to re-target or replace the stylet due to an unacceptable radial error.

The stylet is removed from the peel-away sheath, and the electrode placed to target by inserting it through the sheath. A short scan can be performed to confirm the final location and depth of the electrode. The electrode is then secured by a locking screw and the peel-away sheath removed. We prefer to mark, then secure the Stimloc® clip, as soon as the lead is exposed from the sheath. Then the sheath is fully removed, as is the lead stylet, so the electrode can be removed from the frame and the Stimloc® cap placed. At this point the Smartframe® arc and base can be removed. The end of the lead is capped and buried beneath the scalp as per routine.

Closure and MRI Safety

It is the surgeon's choice whether to obtain a final T1 volumetric scan before or after skin closure. The scan parameters may need to be adjusted to avoid unacceptably high SAR (specific absorption rate) levels once the leads are in place. Your institution's MRI physicist is instrumental in addressing this issue. Unless there is a change in the patient's clinical exam that warrants delayed imaging, this scan can serve as the standard post-operative scan. Performing this scan is not recommended, if performing the procedure in a 3 T scanner [13].

During scalp closure, it is important to recognize that no MRI-compatible suture needles are currently available. This can make suture placement a challenge if the needle is not well-clamped into the needle driver. More importantly, the surgeon and scrub assistant should establish a consistent hand-off routine to prevent a loose needle from flying into the bore. Used needles should be secured in a foam block which is set outside the 5-Gauss line of the magnet. If you use the small screw-driver contained in the Medtronic kit to secure the boot to the proximal lead end, note that this is also ferromagnetic and the same safety concepts must apply.

Intra-operative Pitfalls and Complications

There are aspects of MRI-guided DBS electrode placement that are unique to this modality. As highlighted throughout this chapter, the most important is the need for constant attention to MRI safety. Absent-mindedness can lead to an avoidable injury to the patient or staff. Vigilance ensures a successful and safe procedure.

Also unique to this approach is that the surgeon's view of the brain entry point is reduced at the time of stylet insertion. Therefore, deviation of the stylet caused by bony or dural obstruction at the surface may not be readily identified. Undermining the bony opening and adequate dural opening mitigate this potential pitfall.

Another aspect to take into consideration is the proximity of the mounted bases. This is most relevant in bilateral GPi DBS using a parasagittal approach. Entry points should be planned such that they are at least 5 cm apart from one another to accommodate the bases. Sharply sloping skulls may accommodate shorter distances.

Other pitfalls and risks are similar to any DBS approach. Overall, the complication rate has not been higher than that seen with traditional frame-based implantation methods ([13, 19, 22–24]).

Post-operative Management

Post-operatively, patients should be monitored as per institution standard. Parkinson's medications should be resumed as soon as the patient has recovered sufficiently from anesthesia. If there are no complications or neurologic deficits, the patient can be discharged home on the first or second post-operative day with plan for stage II generator implantation as an outpatient.

Outcomes

In a prospective study of 26 patients who underwent bilateral DBS placement by iMRI using the ClearPoint® System, Ostrem et al. [20] reported a 40.2% improvement in off-medication UPDRS III score at 12 months. This is similar to the outcomes reported in a large series using a standard frame-based approach [7, 25]. Most leads were placed in a single pass ([13, 19, 24]). This may be an advantage of this approach as the number of brain passes may slightly increase the risk for hemorrhage [2, 4].

Overall, the results from these studies are promising, but require a larger patient population and longer follow-up. To date, no study directly comparing outcomes of the iMRI approach to the frame-based approach has been published.

Conclusion

MRI-guided DBS for PD is an evolution of frame-based stereotaxy that has seen significant advancements over the past five years. It is the procedure of choice for Parkinson's patients who cannot tolerate awake DBS placement, but have no contraindications to MR imaging. While it is important to be cognizant of procedure-specific pitfalls, MRI-guided DBS has been shown to have equivalent outcomes to MER-guided DBS placement.

References

1. Amirnovin R, Williams ZM, Cosgrove GR, et al. Experience with microelectrode guided subthalamic nucleus deep brain stimulation. Neurosurgery. 2006;58:ONS96–102.
2. Ben-Haim S, Asaad WF, Gale JT, et al. Risk factors for hemorrhage during microelectrode-guided deep brain stimulation and the introduction of an improved microelectrode design. Neurosurgery. 2009;64:754–62.
3. Benabid AL, Pollak P, Gross C, Hoffmann D, Benazzouz A, Gao DM, et al. Acute and long-term effects of subthalamic nucleus stimulation in Parkinson's disease. Stereotact Funct Neurosurg. 1994;62(1–4):76–84.
4. Binder DK, Rau GM, Starr PA. Risk factors for hemorrhage during microelectrode-guided deep brain stimulator implantation for movement disorders. Neurosurgery. 2005;56:722–32.
5. Brown RA. A computerized tomography-computer graphics approach to stereotaxic localization. J Neurosurg. 1979;50:715–20.

6. Deep brain stimulation for Parkinson's disease study group. Deep brain stimulation of the sub-thalamic nucleus or the pars interna of the globus pallidus in Parkinson's disease. N Engl J Med. 2001;339:1105–11.

7. Deuschl G, Schade-Brittinger C, Krack P, et al. A randomized trial of deep-brain stimulation for Parkinson's disease. N Engl J Med. 2006;355:896–908.

8. Gross RE, Krack P, Rodriguez-Oroz MC, et al. Electrophysiological mapping for the implantation of deep brain stimulators for Parkinson's disease and tremor. Mov Disord. 2006;21:S259–83.

9. Halpern CH, Danish SF, Baltuch GH, et al. Brain shift during deep brain stimulation surgery for Parkinson's disease. Stereotact Funct Neurosurg. 2008;86:37–43.

10. Hariz MI, Fodstad H. Do microelectrode techniques increase accuracy or decrease risks in pallidotomy and deep brain stimulation? A critical review of the literature. Stereotact Funct Neurosurg. 1999;72:157–69.

11. Ivan ME, Yarlagadda J, Saxena AP, et al. Brain shift during bur hole-based procedures using interventional MRI. J Neurosurg. 2014;121:149–60.

12. Khan MF, Mewes K, Gross RE, et al. Assessment of brain shift related to deep brain stimulation surgery. Stereotact Funct Neurosurg. 2008;86:44–53.

13. Larson PS, Richardson RM, Starr PA, et al. Magnetic resonance imaging of implanted deep brain stimulators: experience in a large series. Stereotact Funct Neurosurg. 2008;86:92–100.

14. Larson PS, Starr PA, Bates G, et al. An optimized system for interventional magnetic resonance imaging-guided stereotactic surgery: preliminary evaluation of targeting accuracy. Neurosurgery. 2012;70:S95–103.

15. Larson PS, Starr PA, Martin AJ (version 2.1, updated 2013) Interventional MRI-Guided DBS: A Practical Atlas. An iBook.

16. Martin AJ, Larson PS, Ostrem JL, et al. Placement of deep brain stimulator electrodes using real-time high-field interventional magnetic resonance imaging. Magn Reson Med. 2005;54:1107–14.

17. Martin AJ, Larson PS, Ostrem JL, et al. Interventional magnetic resonance guidance of deep brain stimulator implantation for Parkinson disease. Top Magn Reson Imaging. 2009;19:213–21.

18. McClelland S 3rd, Ford B, Senatus PB, et al. Subthalamic stimulation for Parkinson disease: determination of electrode location necessary for clinical efficacy. Neurosurg Focus. 2005;19:E12.

19. Ostrem JL, Galifianakis NB, Markun LC, Grace JK, Martin AJ, Starr PA, Larson PS. Clinical outcomes of PD patients having bilateral STN DBS using high-field interventional MR-imaging for lead placement. Clin Neurol Neurosurg. 2013;115(6):708–12. https://doi.org/10.1016/j.clineuro.2012.08.019.

20. Ostrem JL, Ziman N, Galifianakis NB, et al. Clinical outcomes using ClearPoint interventional MRI for deep brain stimulation lead placement in Parkinson's disease. J Neurosurg. 2016;124:908–16.

21. Saint-Cyr JA, Hoque T, Pereira LCM, et al. Localization of clinically effective stimulating electrodes in the human subthalamic nucleus on magnetic resonance imaging. J Neurosurg. 2002;97:1152–66.

22. Sidiropoulos C, Rammo R, Merker B, et al. Intraoperative MRI for deep brain stimulation lead placement in Parkinson's disease: 1 year motor and neuropsychological outcomes. J Neurol. 2016;263:1226–31.

23. Starr PA, Markun LC, Larson PS, et al. Interventional MRI-guided deep brain stimulation in pediatric dystonia: first experience with the ClearPoint system. J Neurosurg Pediatr. 2014;14:400–8.

24. Starr PA, Martin AJ, Ostrem JL, et al. Subthalamic nucleus deep brain stimulator placement using high-field interventional magnetic resonance imaging and a skull-mounted aiming device: technique and application accuracy. J Neurosurg. 2010;112:479–90.

25. Weaver F, Follett K, Stern M, et al. Bilateral deep brain stimulation vs best medical therapy for patients with advanced Parkinson disease: a randomized controlled trial. JAMA. 2009;301:63–73.

Optimizing Deep Brain Stimulation Programming in Parkinson's Disease

7

Fiona Gupta and Punit Agrawal

Screening, Expectations, and Assessments

The success of deep brain stimulation (DBS) therapy in Parkinson's disease (PD), whether the target is subthalamic nucleus (STN), globus pallidus interna (GPi), or ventral intermediate thalamus (VIM), starts prior to DBS surgery. The route to best outcomes is based on the proper screening and patient selection, followed by identifying expected clinical benefits and setting the stage with the patient for realistic expectations for goals of DBS therapy.

Screening for DBS candidacy in PD should include movement disorder neurological evaluation, levodopa challenge using a supra-therapeutic dose (if possible), neurosurgical evaluation, cognitive assessment (often with formal neuropsychological testing), possibly a psychiatric assessment and brain imaging.

With the initial evaluation, eliciting the concerns expressed by the patient helps to elucidate the reasons that the patient is seeking DBS therapy. The key elements in the history to suggest benefit for improved quality of life with DBS therapy should include:

1. History of marked response to levodopa, but the development of problematic motor fluctuations with clear problematic/disabling medication off and on time.
2. Medication refractory tremor.
3. Person meeting the diagnostic criteria for diagnosis of idiopathic PD (United Kingdom Brain Bank Criteria).

F. Gupta (✉)
Department of Neurology, The Mount Sinai Hospital, New York, NY, USA
e-mail: fgupta@njbsc.com

P. Agrawal
Department of Neurology and Center for Neuromodulation, The Ohio State University Wexner Medical Center, Columbus, OH, USA

© Springer Nature Switzerland AG 2019
R. R. Goodman (ed.), *Surgery for Parkinson's Disease*,
https://doi.org/10.1007/978-3-319-23693-3_7

Further, if not levodopa intolerant, an important tool in assessing for potential for improvement is a levodopa challenge, by assessing motor symptoms at least 12 h off medications and then after a supra-therapeutic dose of levodopa. In general, medication improvement of PD motor symptoms by greater than 33% tends to indicate a good chance of improving quality of life with DBS therapy, in persons bothered by motor fluctuations.

Importantly, the person's main complaint needs special attention, as it may not be a problem that DBS therapy can be expected to improve. DBS therapy for such a patient may incorrectly be perceived as ineffective. A common practice approach is to re-emphasize the real/expected goals of DBS therapy, in simplistic terms:

1. To reduce motor fluctuations (lessen severity and quantity of off time and lessen dyskinesia).
2. To reduce tremor in individuals with medication refractory tremor.
3. To lessen tremor, bradykinesia, and rigidity in individuals with levodopa intolerance.

Given the nature of the neurodegenerative progression in PD, it is important to highlight which of the above indications is present, and differentiate these from other concerns that tend to not be DBS responsive. Below is a list of some of the specific primary complaints that could be reported during screening and would have little to no expected response to DBS therapy:

1. Gait trouble (such as freezing of gait)
2. Imbalance/falls
3. Posture changes
4. Speech/swallowing trouble
5. Drooling
6. Hypomimia
7. Cognitive issues
8. Bowel/bladder trouble
9. REM sleep disorder
10. Blood pressure fluctuations
11. Non-motor wearing off (i.e. restless legs, fatigue, pain, shortness breath).

When these are the main focus of a patient's concerns, there may be little chance for DBS therapy to improve quality of life.

Also, the specific nature of a patient's bothersome motor symptoms may provide insight into which DBS target will be most beneficial. One example would be a person experiencing return of axial symptoms or gait trouble, when medications wear off, or non-motor symptoms. If these occur in the presence of levodopa-induced dyskinesia, then the GPi target may be considered preferable to STN. GPi DBS also may be preferred over STN in persons with dyskinesia at low doses of levodopa, or when a person is experiencing biphasic dyskinesia. Further, a person predominantly bothered by tremor, without clear motor fluctuations, may see greater benefits from VIM DBS. Especially, this is seen when tremor is mixed with rest, postural, and action components. The selection of the DBS target is important, to achieve successful outcomes and best determined by collaboration of the neurologist and neurosurgeon.

Important information to obtain prior to proceeding with DBS therapy include:

1. Presence of tremor and response to PD medication
2. Amount (hours/minutes) and severity of medication off time with respect to doses of medication, and specific motor symptoms (tremor, rigidity, bradykinesia), with localization to side and part of the body
3. History and details of gait changes with medication wearing off, or if present at peak, response to medications
4. Dyskinesia as it relates to medications: peak effect, presence when medication worn off (such as upon awakening, prior to first morning dose of PD medications), or biphasic with respect to medication onset of action and wearing off
5. Motor score in relationship to best response to medication off/on in a person experiencing motor fluctuations
6. History of levodopa intolerance

These same issues are often useful to reassess at the first visit after DBS therapy has been initiated and kept in mind subsequently, to help identify potential for further improvement with adjustments in DBS parameters and help achieve stimulation optimization.

Patients being screened for DBS commonly need to be educated to understand the meaning of motor symptoms, how to identify off/on time, and to differentiate between dyskinesia and tremor. This education is an important step for future programming visits, and especially given these are the hallmark features for which DBS therapy has likely benefits. In addition, it is very helpful to identify the absence or presence of restless leg syndrome, other non-motor symptoms or dopamine dysregulation syndrome, as these can confound optimization of DBS therapy. The presence of these issues can result in problems with adjusting PD medications, even as clear therapeutic benefits are being achieved with DBS therapy. It is also important to establish if any psychiatric or cognitive issues are present, prior to considering DBS therapy, as these issues commonly interfere with obtaining good DBS outcomes.

With regard to assessing motor symptoms, useful tools include the objective standard rating scales, including Part III of either the UPDRS (United Parkinson's Disease Rating Scale) or MDS-UPDRS (Movement Disorder Society - United Parkinson's Disease Rating Scale). In addition, a person with PD experiencing motor fluctuations may benefit from knowing how to create a motor diary. Another rating scale that can be useful is the UDysRS (Unified Dyskinesia Rating Scale), especially with GPi DBS therapy.

DBS Programming Visits

Basics

At many centers, initiation of DBS therapy for PD patients commonly occurs at 3–4 weeks post-implant of DBS electrode, with subsequent programming visits every 2–6 weeks over the next several months. Maintenance visits thereafter may be every 3–6 months. It can be helpful to reiterate the goals of DBS therapy with each visit.

For the initial programming, it is common practice to use the same examination rating scale that was used preoperatively. This helps identify the absence or presence of a "microlesion" effect (reduced contralateral PD motor symptoms) from DBS lead placement. If present, the "microlesion" effect usually lessens over 1–2 weeks after surgery, but can persist to a milder degree for 6–10 weeks. The continued use of the same rating scale at subsequent visits can also help quantify improvement from prior visits and identify potential for further improvement of off motor symptoms, with further DBS setting changes.

Prior to a programming visit, it is important to establish whether a patient is to come to the visit when medication effects have worn off or during peak effect of a dose of medication. This decision is commonly guided by a person's main concern. If it is the occurrence of off time symptoms (tremor, rigidity, bradykinesia), then programming is best done in the medication off state. If the main concern is dyskinesia, then programming should be done in the medication peak on state. Many DBS Centers find initial and early DBS therapy programming visits most effective in the medication off state (sometimes asking a person to hold 1 dose of PD medication or even not take any PD medications for 12 h). However, this is often individualized based on a programmer preference with regards to the DBS implant site for PD and specific complaints the patient is reporting.

Prior to DBS interrogation/programming, the following history/assessment is commonly helpful:

1. Average daily awake hours of off time and what are the off motor symptoms
2. Average awake hours with dyskinesia and what portion of this time is it bothersome, in addition to what location in the body
3. Continued tremor
4. Possible side effects from stimulation (vide infra)
5. PD medication doses and schedule
6. Objective rating of PD motor symptoms and absence/presence of dyskinesia

Programming

During every programming visit, there is certain basic information that should be reviewed. This includes:

1. Lead model
2. IPG model

3. IPG Battery reading and status
4. % on since last visit
5. Individual monopolar and bipolar electrode impedance (assessing for any open or short circuits)

Adjustable stimulation parameters for DBS include active electrode contacts (for configuration of field), amplitude, pulse width, and frequency.

The mechanism of how DBS induces clinical effects is not well understood. Though stimulation intensity appears to be the key parameter to alleviate symptoms or induce side effects, the other parameters are also important [1–3]. High frequency stimulation (greater than 100 Hz) has been shown to have therapeutic effects and lower frequencies have produced lesser to no clinical effect [1, 2, 4]. Very low frequencies (10 Hz) can worsen symptoms as well [5]. Commonly, DBS therapy is started at 130 Hz and then slowly increased, if needed, but usually not higher than 185 Hz. There is potential for negative effects from stimulation at excessively high frequencies [6]. Pulse width (PW) of 60 and 90 microseconds has been shown to be effective to obtain clinical benefits in PD, thought largely due to activation of large diameter myelinated axons [1]. It is further suspected that lower PW excites large diameter axons and higher PW typically affects smaller diameter and unmyelinated elements [7, 8], thus site of stimulation for therapeutic effect may be different. For example, GPi stimulation may require higher PW than STN or VIM, for therapeutic effects. As a simple rule, an increase in PW tends to make a more concentrated core of stimulation of neuronal elements and may increase therapeutic effects and/or induce unwanted side effects.

Common range of PW and rate in PD based on target:

	Rate (Hertz)	PW (microseconds)
STN	100–185	60–120
GPI	100–130	60–210
VIM	100–185	60–120

The cathode, anode, and amplitude form the stimulation field, with regards to shape and size, and are regarded as the most important parameters for DBS therapy. The field of stimulation is dependent on the location of the implanted electrode with respect to regional anatomy.

Knowledge of the bordering structures and regional anatomy around a nucleus of stimulation, in combination with information of the trajectory and coordinates (relative to the planned target) of the implanted DBS electrode, is instrumental in the selection of the optimal electrode stimulation configuration. Often, a programmer finds reviewing intra-operative notes and related neurophysiological data (if present) helpful as well.

Certain structures around the implanted nucleus are felt to be important, when programming each DBS lead. These structures induce well recognized clinical side effects. In combination with intraoperative records, this can help guide whether the stimulation field should be moved to more dorsal or ventral contacts on the DBS lead (Figs. 7.1, 7.2, and 7.3).

For the STN, posterior stimulation produces persistent paresthesia (medial lemniscus), lateral stimulation produces dystonic muscle contraction/slurred speech/conjugate eye deviation (internal capsule), medial stimulation produces ipsilateral eye deviation/pupil dilatation (cranial nerve III) and flushing/sweating (medial ventral) [9]. In addition, stimulation in the anterior/ventral STN may have no effect or may produce emotional changes.

Fig. 7.1 Axial MRI image at the STN target level, with pertinent structures outlined

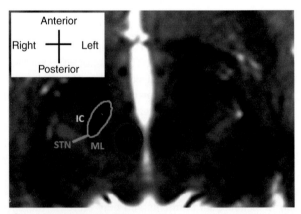

IC = internal capsule
STN = subthalamic nucleus
ML = medial lemniscus
RN = red nucleus

Fig. 7.2 Coronal MRI image at the GPi target level, with pertinent structures outlined

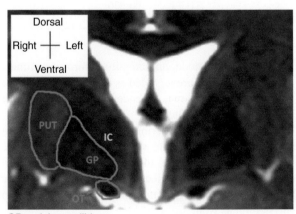

GP = globus pallidus
IC = internal capsule
OT = optic tract
PUT = Putamen

Fig. 7.3 Axial MRI image at the VIM target level, with pertinent structures outlined

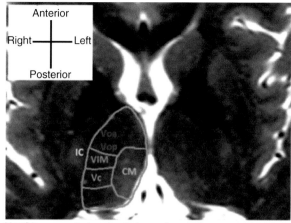

Voa/Vop = ventral oral anterior and posterior
Vim = ventral intermediate
Vc = ventral caudal
IC = internal capsule
CM = central medial

For GPi, medial stimulation can cause dystonic muscle contraction/slurred speech (internal capsule), or visual changes, such as phosphenes (optic tract).

For VIM, the most commonly identified side effects are posterior stimulation, producing persistent paresthesia (Vc – ventral caudal thalamus) and lateral stimulation, causing dystonic muscle contraction/slurred speech (internal capsule).

Thresholds for side effects establish some basic guidelines as to which direction to move the stimulation field, keeping in mind that the electrode trajectory in the brain is from dorsal/anterior/lateral to ventral/posterior/medial.

STN		
Speech change/contraction	Internal capsule	Move medial (more ventral contact)
Ipsilateral eye deviation	Medial	Move lateral (more dorsal contact)
Persistent numbness	Posterior	Move anterior (more dorsal contact)
Sweating/flushing	Medial	Move lateral (more dorsal contact)
GPi		
Phosphenes/visual flashes	Ventral	Move to more dorsal contact
Speech change/contracture	Medial	Move to more dorsal contact
VIM		
Persistent paresthesia	Posterior	Move anterior (more dorsal contact)
Contracture/slurred speech	Lateral	Move medial (more ventral contact)

Programming Specifics

One basic tool commonly referred to during initial and subsequent DBS programming visits is a monopolar review. This will help identify stimulation thresholds by creating a stimulation map in reference to regional anatomical structures and guide selection of stimulation anode (+) and cathode (−). The review is conducted by keeping a constant pulse width (commonly 90 microseconds) and rate (commonly 130 Hertz) and then slowly increasing the amplitude at one electrode contact (cathode) at a time, while using the IPG case as the anode. As the stimulation is increased, clinical observations are made for both evidence of clear symptomatic reduction and, more importantly, the threshold for side effects, due to spread of current to one of the identifiable neighboring structures (recognized by the specific side effect).

The next step is the choice of monopolar or bipolar stimulation, to shape a field of stimulation with the best clinical effect, with the goal of achieving adequate level of clinical benefit, before reaching the threshold for bothersome side effects.

Many DBS programmers will start with monopolar stimulation, but if benefits are suboptimal prior to reaching the stimulation threshold for bothersome side effects, will then switch to bipolar stimulation to try to capture more symptom improvement, before producing bothersome side effects. If two adjacent contacts are found to be effective, a double monopolar configuration can be used to create a larger field (wider and longer). Bipolar stimulation can allow shaping of the field more like a football, thus limiting the width, when side effects occur with the wider field of stimulation. "Near bipolar" uses adjacent contacts and "far bipolar" uses non-adjacent contacts. The most commonly used configurations are as follows (Fig. 7.4):

Other configurations include tripolar or quadripolar, using more than two contacts. If low thresholds for stimulation-induced side effects occur on all electrodes, one useful tripolar configuration is "a guarded cathode" with two anodes surrounding a cathode. These more advanced configurations are rarely used during initial programming visits, but can be tried at future visits, with attempts to improve more clinical symptoms.

During initial programming for STN or GPi DBS, many programmers avoid using frequencies outside of 130–185 Hz or pulse widths outside of 60–100 microseconds, but these should be considered, if needed, at later visits.

With regards to symptoms, the first clinical benefit typically is reduction in rigidity, then tremor, and lastly bradykinesia. Some benefits are seen acutely, but

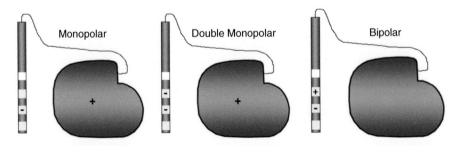

Fig. 7.4 Schematic diagrams depicting different modes of stimulation

there is usually further reduction over several minutes to hours and even further reduction is often seen over the next few weeks. With STN DBS therapy, dyskinesia may occur with effective stimulation therapy, after a few minutes or a few hours. This will often worsen with doses of medication. An increase in dyskinesia can be alleviated by a combination of medication reduction and lowering of stimulation. This is then followed by a gradual increase of stimulation over the next several weeks. To lessen the chance of dyskinesia, some programmers will adjust parameters until clinical benefits are seen and then lower the stimulation at the end of the visit. This approach will be followed by visits to slowly increase stimulation parameters, in addition to possible medication adjustments. Another strategy that can be employed is increasing stimulation to effective parameters, and then immediately cutting PD medications at the end of the visit, with caution to not induce withdrawal side effects from too rapid of a reduction. Regardless of a programmer's preference, it is often very useful to observe a patient after taking a dose of PD medications and see the full on effect, in case further adjustments are needed, due to on side effects. This is of particular importance during the initial programming visit. Every programmer has different strategies, and these may vary from patient to patient.

Newer DBS Leads

Recently, newer DBS lead models have become available. Two specific features of interest include electrode segmentation and fractionalization. These features may not be needed for many patients, but allow for flexibility for finer tuning. These are most helpful when there is need to further shape the field of stimulation, due to a low threshold for side effects.

A segmented lead has the middle two of the four electrodes divided into three. This provides a total of 8 possible stimulation electrodes instead of 4, and allows for a stimulation field to be shaped away from a neighboring structure causing lower threshold for side effects. A fractionalized lead allows for any of the electrodes to be used with any percentile of the total energy. This also allows shaping the stimulation field to avoid unwanted side effects. Other investigations are ongoing to further explore the full potential of these leads.

References

1. Rizzone M, et al. Deep brain stimulation of the subthalamic nucleus in Parkinson's disease: effects of variation in stimulation parameters. J Neurol Neurosurg Psychiatry. 2001;71:215–9.
2. Moro E, et al. The impact on Parkinson's disease of electrical parameter settings in STN stimulation. Neurology. 2002;59:706–13.
3. Dayal V, et al. Subthalamic nucleus deep brain stimulation in Parkinson's disease: the effect of varying stimulation parameters. J Parkinsons Dis. 2017;7:235–45.
4. Limousin P, et al. Effect of parkinsonian signs and symptoms of bilateral subthalamic nucleus stimulation. Lancet. 1995;345:91–5.

5. Timmerman L, et al. Ten hertz stimulation of the subthalamic nucleus deteriorates motor symptoms in Parkinson's disease. Mov Disord. 2004;19:1328–33.
6. Limousin P, et al. Abnormal involuntary movements induced by subthalamic nucleus stimulation in parkinsonian patients. Mov Disord. 1996;11:231–5.
7. McIntyre C, et al. Cellular effects of deep brain stimulation: model-based analysis of activation and inhibition. J Neurophysiol. 2004;91:1457–69.
8. Ranck J. Which elements are excited in electrical stimulation of mammalian central nervous system: a review. Brain Res. 1975;98:417–40.
9. Krack P, et al. Postoperative management of subthalamic nucleus stimulation for Parkinson's disease. Mov Disord. 2002;17(Suppl. 3):S188–97.

DBS Revision Surgery: Indications and Nuances

David Shin, Justin D. Hilliard, and Kelly D. Foote

Introduction

Deep brain stimulation surgery has become the treatment of choice for appropriately selected patients with Parkinson's disease, essential tremor, and dystonia. Despite the significant risk associated with minimally invasive brain surgery, the risk-to-benefit ratio for DBS surgery is quite favorable, and the overwhelming majority of patients derive substantial improvement in their motor function and quality of life from well-executed DBS therapy. A nonnegligible number of movement disorders patients, however, report unsatisfactory outcomes after DBS surgery. If we define *"DBS failure"* as any case in which the patient and her/his caregivers are dissatisfied with the outcome of DBS surgery, then potential causes of DBS failure include failure to set appropriate expectations preoperatively, inappropriate patient selection, failures of postoperative device programming and medical management, in addition to various surgical and device-related complications including suboptimal lead placement, hardware failures, and rare instances of procedure-related brain injury resulting in permanent neurologic impairment. In one published series of 41 consecutive patients who presented for evaluation of DBS failure, approximately half of the failures were attributable to surgical and device-related complications [1]. Forty-six percent of patients had suboptimally positioned DBS leads in that series [1]. Other reported surgically remediable causes of DBS failure are less common, and include infection, skin erosion, pulse generator battery depletion, and DBS lead or extension fractures [2–6]. At the University of Florida, our team has evaluated over 400 patients referred to our center for DBS failure and we have performed over 100 surgical procedures aimed at remediating these cases. Just over half of these referred patients were converted from patient-defined DBS failures to successes with various interventions. Fortunately, with

D. Shin · J. D. Hilliard · K. D. Foote (✉)
University of Florida, Department of Neurosurgery, Gainesville, FL, USA
e-mail: foote@neurosurgery.ufl.edu

© Springer Nature Switzerland AG 2019
R. R. Goodman (ed.), *Surgery for Parkinson's Disease*,
https://doi.org/10.1007/978-3-319-23693-3_8

careful patient screening and appropriate surgical intervention, a high percentage of the patients who ultimately underwent DBS revision surgery derived substantial benefit from it [1, 2, 7–9]. In this chapter, we focus on the various causes of DBS failure that are potentially correctable through surgical intervention. We review methods for evaluating patients presenting with DBS failure to identify appropriate candidates for various surgical salvage procedures, and we present successful decision-making strategies and surgical techniques for carrying out these operations.

Multidisciplinary Risk-Benefit Analysis

Perhaps, even more so than for initial DBS surgery, the decision to perform DBS revision surgery warrants a very careful *analysis of the patient-specific risks and predictable benefits* associated with repeat surgical intervention. Because failure to achieve predicted efficacy of DBS therapy, or delayed loss of efficacy, may be attributable to a variety of factors, we find it useful in our decision-making process to obtain input from a *multidisciplinary team* qualified to examine all facets of a patient's disease, surgical intervention, and outcomes. At our center, patients presenting with "DBS failure" (like patients referred for initial DBS surgery) are evaluated by a team of *eight different specialists*, all of whom are subspecialized in movement disorders, and all of whom have evaluated hundreds of patients prior to and after DBS surgery. The initial evaluation is performed by a movement disorders neurologist who serves as gatekeeper for the interdisciplinary evaluation. If the neurologist determines, on initial screening, that the patient was likely an appropriate candidate for DBS surgery and that the predicted benefits of DBS therapy were not realized, she/he refers the patient for a 2-day risk/benefit analysis that includes evaluations by the following specialists: DBS surgeon, neuropsychologist, psychiatrist, physical therapist (PT), occupational therapist (OT), speech/swallow disorders specialist, and social worker. The neurologist's extensive initial evaluation includes confirmation of the patient's neurologic diagnosis, review of the patient's history and previous response to pertinent medication trials, evaluation of the patient's symptom severity and responses to both medical and DBS therapy (e.g., assessing UPDRS motor score in various states: Off-medication/Off-stimulation, Off-med/On-stim, On-med/Off-stim, On-med/On-stim), assessing responses to adjustment of medications and/or stimulation parameters including assessment of the electrical integrity of the DBS system and documentation of thresholds for stimulation-induced side effects at each DBS contact, and brain imaging (MRI +/− high-resolution CT) for careful anatomic localization of the existing DBS lead(s). In one series of patients referred to two academic centers for DBS failure, 12% were subsequently diagnosed with a neurologic disorder not typically expected to respond well to DBS therapy [1]. The various other specialists involved in the decision-making process each assess the patient-specific risks and potential benefits of further surgical intervention within their specialized domain based upon extensive prior experience with similar patients. For example, increased risk of further surgery may be discovered by PT (poor balance/fall risk), speech therapy (dysarthria, aspiration), psychiatry (depression, anxiety disorder), neuropsychology (poor cognitive reserve, dysfluent speech), or neurosurgery (advanced age, severe brain atrophy, multiple medical comorbidities). Alternatively, the OT might point out that the right brain DBS lead in an essential tremor patient who reports no significant improvement in her dominant left-hand tremor after initial DBS surgery seems poorly positioned and has excessively low thresholds for stimulation-induced side effects, rendering it essentially useless. The social worker adds that the patient must be able to feed herself in order to stay in the assisted living center that she loves, joining with the OT to make a compelling argument that replacement of the poorly placed right DBS lead would likely result in a very meaningful improvement in the patient's functioning and quality of life.

Nonsurgically Remediable Reasons for DBS Failure

Over half of all patients who present with DBS failure have problems that cannot be remedied with surgical intervention, but DBS surgeons should be keenly aware of these problems and should play a key role in their prevention. In the worst of cases, a patient presents with a bad outcome that was predictable because she/he was a poor candidate for DBS surgery in the first place. In such cases, careful screening with an experienced multidisciplinary team would likely have led to a consensus recommendation against surgery due to perceived risks that clearly outweighed predictable benefits. In some cases, both patient selection and surgical procedure are well executed, but suboptimal postoperative management results in patient dissatisfaction. In many such cases, DBS programming and medication adjustments can salvage a good outcome. Occasionally, appropriate patient selection, along with sound surgical and postoperative management, results in predictable symptomatic improvement with minimal adverse effects, but patients and caregivers are dissatisfied because their expectations were unrealistic and the failure was one of preoperative education. In such cases, extensive counseling with the patient and caregivers, along with multidisciplinary optimization of care, typically results in a reasonable level of restored satisfaction.

Surgically Remediable Reasons for DBS Failure

Hardware Failure

Damage to a DBS lead or extension cable is often discovered after a sudden loss of clinical efficacy, or when an intermittent shocking sensation is felt by the patient [5, 10–12]. Interrogation of the pulse generator revealing elevated impedance on one or more contacts suggests an open circuit consistent with *lead fracture*. Similarly, damage to a lead or extension can result in a *short circuit* between two contacts, resulting in low impedance measurements over the bipolar circuit in question and identical impedance measurements when the affected circuits are tested against the case, in monopolar mode. Commonly, only a single contact is affected by lead fracture. If the contact affected by the lead fracture is the active contact and therapeutic efficacy is lost, *reprogramming* is performed in an attempt to use surrounding viable contacts to salvage therapeutic benefit.

If reprogramming fails to restore acceptable clinical efficacy, then surgical intervention is indicated. An X-ray series (skull and chest) capturing the course of the electrode, extension cable, and IPG should be performed prior to surgery in an attempt to localize the malfunctioning hardware component. Most commonly, short circuits and open circuits involving only a subset of the DBS contacts do not result in a visible discontinuity in the lead or extension cable on X-ray. Occasionally, however, a significant disruption of the integrity of the lead or extension might be identifiable on X-rays, facilitating planned surgical correction of the problem. When the site of the hardware failure is indeterminate, which is most commonly the case, our strategy is to *replace the extension cable (and the generator if it is nearing the end of its battery life),* in an outpatient procedure, in an attempt to solve the problem without replacing the intracranial lead, which would be substantially more invasive and expensive. In our experience with the most commonly used DBS hardware system, the pulse generator is almost never the source of a hardware failure unless it is nearing end of life. The integrity of the intracranial lead can be tested independently during the extension replacement procedure, but the reliability of this testing is not perfect and we typically attribute an open or short circuit to a damaged lead, if replacement of the extension cable does not restore the electrical integrity of the system. The patient should be well informed regarding the possibility that replacement of the extension cable and the pulse generator might not solve the problem, and that if the problem lies with the intracranial DBS lead, then this can only be corrected with a stereotactic cranial procedure to remove and replace the lead. In our experience using our current DBS implantation techniques, the intracranial lead is rarely the source of a hardware failure and replacement of the extension generally resolves the problem. Multiple *technical modifications have diminished the incidence of DBS lead fracture* in our experience. These include the following: (1) avoiding placement of the *connector in the neck* as repetitive neck movement can result, over time, in fatigue and fracture of the lead at its junction with the rigid connector; (2) careful application of *pinching counter-torque* to each individual metal block in the connector as its connection is tightened can prevent rotation of the block within the polymer casing that may result in shearing of the individual wires and open circuits; (3) avoidance of excessive *tensile force applied to the "dummy connector"* attached to the implanted lead prior to its connection to the extension cable, which can result in fracture of the most vulnerable #3 circuit wire near its attachment to the connection contact; (4) avoiding the application of any significant *tensile force on the segment of the lead where contacts are distributed*, which can result in detachment of the bond between the polymer casing and the contacts with stretching and exposure of the internal helically coiled wires and potential fractures and open circuits; and (5) taking care to *align the connection contacts with their blocks prior to tightening* the connection screws, since tightening the connection screws onto an interval of polymer encased lead rather than onto the intended metal contacts can result in damage to the polymer insulation surrounding individual wires, producing short circuits.

First described in individual's with cardiac pacemakers [13], *twiddler's syndrome* is defined as manipulation of the IPG resulting in hardware failure. Twiddler's syndrome more commonly occurs in patients who are obese or in women with pendulous breasts. In such patients, more abundant subcutaneous adipose tissue allows the implanted pulse generator to more easily rotate. Repetitive rotation of the IPG results in twisting of the extension cables that can result in tension, fracture, or, in extreme cases, lead migration. We have also seen twiddling in nonobese patients with connective tissue disorders or psychiatric disorders. Revision surgery to securely anchor the pulse generator in place may be performed to avoid the sequelae of twiddler's syndrome. One may even consider subpectoral placement of the IPG with silk suture anchors to prevent IPG rotation. Subpectoral placement is not feasible for rechargeable devices, however, because the increased depth of implantation would prevent recharging [4, 14–16].

Because of the more significant risk associated with lead replacement, *the intracranial lead should only be replaced after ruling out extension cable or IPG malfunction*. A careful risk/benefit analysis should be undertaken prior to lead replacement surgery, because a patient with acceptable risk for cranial surgery may transition into a patient with unacceptable risk as aging and predictable disease progression result in diminished physiologic reserve.

Lead Migration

Post-implantation lead migration may occur for a variety of reasons. Methods for securing DBS leads at their point of egress from the skull vary among surgeons. The most common technique uses the Stimloc cap supplied by Medtronic. The point of fixation during closure of the "Pac-man"- type locking mechanism is weak, offering minimal resistance to tensile or compressive axial forces. Great care must be taken during securing the lead with this cap, not to inadvertently advance the lead deeper or pull the lead out. After multiple episodes of inadvertent *intraoperative dorsal lead migration* in our early experience at the University of Florida, we adopted the use of intraoperative fluoroscopy to ensure that the leads are not displaced during the fixation process.

We have also learned, through careful analysis of our own technical errors over time, that even the fully assembled Stimloc cap has insufficient strength to withstand a significant tensile force, which can result in *dorsal lead migration postoperatively*. During staged pulse generator implantation, the most commonly used DBS system requires exposure of approximately 4 cm of the previously implanted DBS lead in order to place a connection cover and connect the new extension cable to the previously implanted DBS lead. This is typically accomplished by making a small scalp incision over the proximal aspect of the palpable "dummy connector" on the "connection" end of the implanted DBS lead and pulling on the lead to expose a sufficient length of the lead to make the connection to a newly tunneled cable. Following a series of unexplained dorsal lead migrations over the course of a few years, we performed a study to determine the incidence and etiology of postoperative dorsal lead migration. In a series of 135 cases in which patients had undergone high-resolution CT imaging enabling precise measurement of the position of an implanted DBS lead (or leads) on at least two occasions separated in time by at least 3 months, 12% of patients were found to have dorsal migration of their DBS leads by greater than 3 mm. Multiple hypotheses were proposed and investigated to explain this observation, and ultimately it became compellingly clear that all of the dorsal lead migrations were attributable to excessive coaxial tensile force applied to the lead and failure of the cap fixation at the skull. Most commonly, this was attributable to poor surgical technique with application of excessive tension during connection of the lead to the extension cable. When the interval between lead implantation and pulse generator implantation exceeds 3 weeks, the lead becomes sufficiently scarred into the subgaleal space that the applied tensile force, rather than resulting in pulling out a coiled loop of subgaleal lead, is transmitted coaxially along the scarred in lead, resulting in some cases in failure of the lead fixation point at the Stimloc cap and withdrawal of the lead from the brain. (Fig. 8.1) In rare cases (head movement due to dystonia, twiddler's syndrome), tensile forces exerted by the patient resulted in similar fixation failure and dorsal lead migration. (Unpublished manuscript in preparation.) In another published retrospective review of 240 electrodes, 7.9% of dystonia patients experienced migration of their lead, while there were no migrations found in PD, MS, or tremor patients. The predisposition for dystonia patients to experience lead migration is presumed to be attributable to their extensive head and neck movements imposing significant strain on their intracranial and extension cables [12].

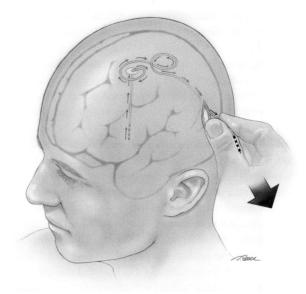

Fig. 8.1 This illustration shows the tensor force transmitted from the dummy connector to the tip of the electrode inside of the brain, resulting in iatrogenic dorsal lead migration

Intraoperative lead migration can be effectively prevented by carefully avoiding inadvertent pulling on the lead, while it is being secured to the skull after implantation, and by comparing intraoperative fluoroscopic images before and after lead fixation to ensure that no displacement has occurred during fixation.

In order to prevent postoperative lead migration, we have adopted the strategy of making a longer incision coaxially proximal to and along the palpable subgaleal dummy connector and minimizing tensile force applied to expose sufficient lead for the connection. We also drill recesses in the skull at the Stimloc and the connector sites to minimize the prominence of the implanted hardware. This effectively prevents delayed scalp erosions (unpublished manuscript in preparation), but also mitigates the transmission of a coaxial tensile force from the extension cable to the lead, which should diminish the likelihood of dorsal lead migration secondary to twiddling or dystonic movements.

In the event of loss of DBS efficacy due to a dorsal lead migration that is confirmed by imaging and careful lead localization, programming at more ventral contacts should be attempted prior to surgical revision of the lead. If this is unsuccessful, the lead should be removed and replaced with a new lead. *Attempts at advancing the lead to a deeper position beyond the early postoperative period are rarely successful* due to removal of the stiffening stylet and softening of the implanted lead that occurs over time, at body temperature.

Suboptimal Lead Position

Suboptimal lead location may be attributable to the use of indirect targeting, head movement or frame shift, excessive CSF loss intraoperatively resulting in brain shift, or postoperative lead migration. Given that the targets for DBS are on a subcentimeter scale, a difference in lead position of a few millimeters can make the difference between effective symptom relief and intolerable side effects [2].

In our first study on DBS failure in 2005, 19 of 41 patients had suboptimally positioned DBS leads, and poor lead placement continues to be a contributing factor in roughly half of all DBS failure patients referred to our center [1]. Interestingly, we only perform lead replacement surgery in about half of the patients in whom a DBS lead is determined to be suboptimally positioned. This discrepancy is largely attributable to the multidisciplinary risk/benefit analysis described above. When the risk of further surgical intervention is determined to exceed the expected benefit from such intervention (not an uncommon occurrence), then a consensus recommendation is made against further surgical intervention.

No amount of expert programming can compensate for a poorly placed DBS lead. Decreasing the likelihood of suboptimal lead placement is of paramount importance for a surgical procedure in which a millimeter or two can determine the difference between remarkable symptomatic relief with profound patient satisfaction and a procedure that fails to achieve its only goal of enhancing quality of life, because stimulation-induced side effects outweigh clinical benefits.

We advocate the use of high-resolution, 3 Tesla gadolinium-enhanced T1-MPRAGE and FGATIR MRI coupled with a deformable, patient-specific three-dimensional atlas to enable careful direct targeting of the DBS lead [17]. Using software capable of displaying the position of the DBS lead within the 3D virtual representation of the brain, a safe trajectory can be selected for each patient (avoiding surface and periventricular veins, ependymal surfaces, sulci, and deep vessels), and the position of the DBS contacts within the target can be visualized and adjusted with small alterations of the target and trajectory to customize targeting to each patient's brain (i.e., *direct targeting*).

In addition to careful stereotactic targeting, *intraoperative physiologic and radiographic feedback* can be exploited to optimize outcomes. While the value of intraoperative *microelectrode recording* has become controversial, we remain convinced that skillful MER can provide useful fine-tuning of the anatomic target that warrants the small associated risk. Similarly, as patient-friendly, purely anatomically targeted "asleep DBS" methods using intraoperative imaging are becoming more prevalent, the importance of assessing thresholds for stimulation-induced side effects and evaluating clinical benefit intraoperatively using *trial stimulation* via *the implanted DBS lead* has been questioned. To date, our group remains unconvinced that DBS targeting with imaging alone (even the very high-quality 3T MR imaging described above—let alone the far less optimal imaging that is typically achievable intraoperatively) is superior to methods that augment image-guided targeting with physiologic feedback. It is likely that experienced DBS practitioners will achieve a high percentage of good outcomes using only image-based targeting, but it also seems likely that foregoing intraoperative test stimulation via the implanted DBS lead will result in some, hopefully slight, increase in the number of patients with DBS failure attributable to intolerable stimulation-induced side effects that occur before predicted therapeutic benefit can be achieved. Our philosophy that *neither safety nor efficacy should be compromised for the sake of convenience* has led us to continue to use awake surgery with physiologic feedback for the overwhelming majority of our patients.

A critical step in the evaluation of a patient with DBS failure is *accurate anatomical localization of the existing DBS lead*. We contend that every implanted DBS lead should be carefully localized postoperatively for quality control and to assist with programming. At our center, each DBS patient undergoes a high-resolution head CT for lead localization approximately 3–4 weeks after the lead implantation procedure. For convenience, this CT is acquired systematically as part of the preoperative evaluation the day prior to initial pulse generator implantation. The postoperative CT is fused to the preoperative targeting 3 T MRI and patient-specific three-dimensional atlas. The delayed acquisition of the lead localization CT allows the resolution of any pneumocephalus and brain shift caused by the lead implantation procedure and results in a higher fidelity image fusion. The position of the DBS contacts are carefully measured on the high-resolution CT (more accurate than MRI for determining the precise position of the lead) and the lead is displayed graphically on the fused MRI/atlas. This enables prediction of which DBS contact is likely to be most favorably positioned for therapeutic stimulation and can facilitate DBS programming. For patients referred from other centers, we use a similar protocol with 1.5 Tesla MRI (MPRAGE+gadolinium and FGATIR) and a patient-specific 3D atlas (+/− high-resolution postoperative CT) to localize the lead anatomically [17].

The *lead localization* thus performed is used in conjunction with the *thresholds for stimulation-induced side effects* measured for each contact and an assessment of *clinical benefit* (or lack thereof) achieved with optimally programmed stimulation *to determine whether the lead is poorly placed.* For example, a patient with debilitating essential tremor presents after DBS surgery complaining that she can only achieve meaningful tremor suppression at high voltage settings, but these settings result in intolerably dysarthric speech and swallowing difficulty. Lead localization shows that the DBS contacts are positioned on the boundary between the VIM thalamus and the internal capsule. The determination is made that the existing DBS lead is positioned excessively lateral, and that if the perceived risks are acceptable, then removal and replacement of the lead to a position 2.5–3 mm more medial would likely result in diminished side effects and substantial improvement of her tremor suppression (and her satisfaction) with DBS therapy. A detailed understanding of the typical DBS targets and their surrounding anatomy is critical to this decision-making process. Understanding which stimulation-induced side effects result from the spreading of current into which neurocircuitry surrounding the target enables the astute DBS practitioner to plan effective lead repositioning procedures when indicated (Table 8.1).

Table 8.1 Typical stimulation-induced side effects and their anatomic correlates

Side effect	Electrode positioning in STN
Muscular contraction	Lateral or anterior (internal capsule)
Paraesthesias	Posterior or medial (medial lemniscus)
Autonomic symptoms (flushing, sweating)	Anterior or medial
Diplopia	Medial (CN III)
Dysarthria	Lateral or anterior (internal capsule)
Personality or impulsivity changes	Medial or ventral (SNr)
Side effect	Electrode positioning in GPI
Muscular contraction	Posterior or medial (internal capsule)
Flashes of light	Ventral
No effect	Lateral, superior, or anterior
Side effect	Electrode positioning in VIM
Muscular contraction	Lateral (internal capsule)
Dysarthria/dysphagia	Lateral and anterior (internal capsule/corticobulbar)
Limbic effects (mania, anxiety)	Medial

Strategies for Surgical Rescue of DBS Failures

DBS Lead Replacement

In cases where minimal to no therapeutic benefit is derived from DBS therapy despite valiant and expert programming, no evidence of hardware failure is present, and careful anatomic and physiologic localization of the lead (as described above) confirms an obviously suboptimal lead position, the decision to remove the poorly placed lead and implant a new lead is relatively straightforward [2]. In general, lead replacement should not be undertaken unless the ineffective lead is at least 2 mm away from the planned reimplantation site. The planned reimplantation site should be selected preoperatively to correct apparent anatomic misplacement that is confirmed with predictable stimulation-induced adverse effects. After performing over 50 lead replacement procedures, we have identified two common misconceptions regarding DBS lead replacement surgery: (1) Contrary to popular belief, *the risk of removal of a DBS lead, regardless of how long it has been implanted, is minimal*. We have never encountered significant adherence of the implanted lead to the brain or caused a hemorrhage or stroke by removing a chronically implanted DBS lead. Every lead we have removed has slid out of the brain with essentially no resistance; (2) *It is not necessary to perform independent, staged procedures to remove a DBS lead then place a new one*. As long as the new target is at least a couple of millimeters away from the old one, the risk of reimplanting into the exact same (ineffective) location is minimal, brain shift is not a major issue, and microelectrode recording at the new implantation site is not adversely effected.

Unless the existing entry site is suboptimal due to safety concerns for the new trajectory (prominent cortical veins, crossing ependymal surfaces, etc.) *we generally try to use the existing entry site* to implant the replacement lead to avoid creating new, independent penetration pathways through the brain. In most cases, skull bone has regenerated to at least partially fill the previous burr hole, so even if the same entry site is planned, the burr hole requires some drilling. If the existing Stimloc cap is attached to the outer cortex of the skull and produces a prominence on the patient's head, we replace the existing Stimloc entirely and take advantage of the opportunity to *drill a recess in the skull to countersink the cap and make it flush with the surrounding skull*. If the cap is already countersunk, we might leave the base ring in place and replace only the snap in "Pac-man" mechanism and the overlying cover. The surgical procedure employed for lead replacement is otherwise essentially identical to that for original lead implantation, with the exception that we generally try to connect the new lead to the existing extension cable at the end of the procedure, rather than coming back for a second stage to connect the new lead.

In the case series mentioned above that evaluated patients referred for "DBS failure," 46% (19 of 41) were deemed to have poorly placed electrodes with 24% (10 of 41) proceeding to surgical replacement of their DBS leads [1]. Of those who underwent surgical revision, 70% experienced marked improvement, while 30%

experienced partial improvement. Fifty-one percent (21 of 41) of patients who were referred for DBS failure ultimately had good outcomes with alteration of their medical regimen or due to surgical revision, 15% (6 of 41) had modest improvement, and 34% (14 of 41) did not improve [1].

Addition of a "Rescue Lead"

In DBS cases where patients experience some clinical improvement that is meaningful, but substantially less than that predicted preoperatively, and lead localization does not clearly suggest a poorly positioned lead, the decision-making regarding further surgery is less straightforward. In such cases, removal of the existing DBS lead might result in loss of the meaningful, but limited therapeutic benefit from the original lead with no guarantee that a new lead would be an improvement. In such cases, if we are convinced that there is potential for substantial symptomatic improvement, and the risk/benefit ratio is appropriate, we generally opt to leave the partially effective lead in place and carefully implant an additional "rescue" lead through a separate entry site into an alternative target that would be expected to provide synergistic benefit. There is limited literature regarding the overall effectiveness of rescue leads, but several case reports and a case series have indicated that rescue leads are a potentially effective method of management of partial DBS failure [7–9, 18].

The following are examples of successful application of this rescue lead strategy:

1. Addition of *GPi rescue leads to suppress problematic dyskinesia* in a patient with traditional STN DBS for Parkinson's disease who continues to derive significant relief of bradykinesia, rigidity, and tremor, but has developed problematic dyskinesia over time. The very reliable dyskinesia suppression achievable with GPi DBS makes this an excellent strategy for such patients.
2. Addition of an *additional GPi rescue lead in the ipsilateral GPi nucleus of a patient with incompletely relieved dystonia* and an apparently reasonable, but suboptimally positioned GPi lead. (The motor segment of the GPi is a considerably larger target than that of the STN, and higher current delivery is typically required to achieve desired stimulation effects as compared to the significantly smaller STN, and hence the observed longer battery lives associated with STN stimulation.) In such a situation, a second lead within the same nucleus may be warranted in order to provide additional benefit. An example of such a strategy was documented in the case series by Oyama et al. [8], in which a patient with cervical dystonia initially underwent bilateral GPi implantation but experienced only pain relief without a substantial improvement in her UDRS score (reduced from 11 to 10). Imaging revealed that her leads were within the GPi, but that her left lead was 2.4 mm more anterior than the right lead. A rescue lead was placed more posteriorly on the left, after which her UDRS score improved to 4.

3. *Addition of an ipsilateral STN (or caudal zona incerta) DBS lead in a patient with meaningful, but incomplete suppression of debilitating essential tremor* with traditional VIM thalamic stimulation.
4. *Addition of bilateral STN stimulators in a patient with severe generalized torsion dystonia who has incompletely responded to traditional bilateral GPi stimulation.*
5. *Addition of bilateral GPi stimulators in a patient with incomplete relief of severe Parkinsonian symptoms with bilateral STN stimulation.* This strategy was employed successfully by Allert et al. [18] for a PD patient who underwent bilateral STN DBS that initially improved her off-medication UPDRS score from 83 to 31. Over several years, her disease progressed and her DBS became less effective, resulting in worsening of her off-medication UPDRS score closer to her preoperative baseline, at 78. She underwent additional bilateral GPi DBS implantation that reduced her off-med UPDRS score to 47.
6. *Addition of a* ventral oralis *(VO) DBS lead in a patient with incomplete suppression of severe tremor with traditional VIM stimulation.* Oyama et al. [8] reported such an essential tremor patient who underwent VIM implantation at another institution with meaningful improvement, but continued significant tremor with a TRS score of 28. He underwent addition of a VO DBS lead, which improved his tremor and reduced his TRS to 17. We have had gratifying success with a dual lead ipsilateral (VIM + VO) thalamic DBS technique for suppression of very severe tremor, and we have adopted the strategy—for patients with very severe tremor—of implanting a VIM DBS lead, testing intraoperatively, and if the tremor suppression achieved with test stimulation through the VIM lead is not satisfactory, we will immediately add a second lead in the ipsilateral VO nucleus.
7. *Addition of an ipsilateral GPi DBS rescue lead to treat iatrogenic hemiballismus in a patient who suffered a rare delayed STN infarct 1 year after implantation of clinically effective STN DBS.* Oyama et al. [9] reported a patient treated with bilateral STN DBS for PD who developed hemiballismus, believed to have occurred as a result of a small STN stroke secondary to lead placement. This patient underwent implantation of an ipsilateral GPi rescue lead, which successfully suppressed his hemiballismus.

Programming of rescue leads will depend on the extent of benefit obtained when both leads are active versus isolated stimulation of the rescue lead. In the majority of cases in which the patient is already experiencing some benefit from his original lead, multi-lead stimulation results in maximum symptomatic relief. If patients are found to have equivalent benefit without activation of the original lead, then single lead stimulation may be a more effective strategy, especially in Parkinson's disease, where studies have demonstrated that dual stimulation of GPi and STN does not necessarily provide synergistic benefit [19, 20]. Patients deemed candidates for rescue leads should be thoroughly evaluated by a multidisciplinary team in order to carefully weigh the benefits and risks of additional lead placement.

Conclusion

DBS has become a mature and reliable therapy for the treatment of debilitating, medication refractory movement disorders. By exploiting our collective experience and available outcomes data, we should be able to reliably identify patients who are likely to benefit from DBS therapy and make accurate predictions regarding which of their presenting symptoms are likely to improve and by approximately how much. When individual patient outcomes after DBS surgery fall short of our predictions, patients and caregivers are understandably dissatisfied. Since DBS is not a lifesaving or curative procedure, and the sole objective of DBS therapy is to improve quality of life, when this goal is not met, the designation of such cases as "DBS Failures" is not overly harsh. Careful, systematic troubleshooting of cases of DBS failure, including evaluation by a multidisciplinary team of movement disorders specialists, accurate localization of the ineffective DBS lead, interrogation of the DBS system to rule out hardware failure, and a trial of expert programming of the existing lead, can typically identify the cause(s) of DBS failure. Causes can be divided into surgically remediable and nonsurgically remediable. Problems that are not amenable to surgical intervention include poor patient selection, failure to exploit a multidisciplinary team to appropriately predict risk versus benefit of surgical intervention, poor perioperative management of medications, ineffective programming, and failure to set appropriate patient and/or caregiver expectations. Surgically remediable DBS failures include hardware failure, lead migration, suboptimal lead position, skin/scalp erosion, and infection. In this chapter, we reviewed techniques for avoiding such failures and discussed useful strategies for management of surgically correctable DBS failures, such as DBS lead replacement and addition of rescue DBS leads, with detailed explanation of the technical aspects of these interventions.

References

1. Okun MS, Tagliati M, Pourfar M, Fernandez HH, Rodriguez RL, Alterman RL, et al. Management of referred deep brain stimulation failures: a retrospective analysis from 2 movement disorders centers. Arch Neurol. 2005;62:1250–5.
2. Ellis TM, Foote KD, Fernandez HH, Sudhyadhom A, Rodriguez RL, Zeilman P, et al. Reoperation for suboptimal outcomes after deep brain stimulation surgery. Neurosurgery. 2008;63:754–60 discussion 760-751.
3. Falowski SM, Ooi YC, Bakay RA. Long-term evaluation of changes in operative technique and hardware-related complications with deep brain stimulation. Neuromodulation. 2015;18(8):670–7.
4. Guridi J, Rodriguez-Oroz MC, Alegre M, Obeso JA. Hardware complications in deep brain stimulation: electrode impedance and loss of clinical benefit. Parkinsonism Relat Disord. 2012;18:765–9.
5. Morishita T, Foote KD, Burdick AP, Katayama Y, Yamamoto T, Frucht SJ, Okun MS. Identification and management of deep brain stimulation intra- and postoperative urgencies and emergencies. Parkinsonism Relat Disord. 2010;16:153–62.
6. Troche MS, Brandimore AE, Foote KD, Okun MS. Swallowing and deep brain stimulation in Parkinson's disease: a systematic review. Parkinsonism Relat Disord. 2013;19:783–8.

7. Matias CM, Silva D, Machado AG, Cooper SE. Rescue of bilateral subthalamic stimulation by bilateral pallidal stimulation: case report. J Neurosurg. 2016;124(2):417–21.
8. Oyama G, Foote KD, Hwynn N, Jacobson CE, Malaty IA, Rodriguez RL, et al. Rescue leads: a salvage technique for selected patients with a suboptimal response to standard DBS therapy. Parkinsonism Relat Disord. 2011;17:451–5.
9. Oyama G, Maling N, Avila-Thompson A, Zeilman PR, Foote KD, Malaty IA, Rodriguez RL, Okun MS. Rescue GPi-DBS for a stroke-associated hemiballism in a patient with STN-DBS. Tremor Other Hyperkinet Mov (N Y). 2014;4:tre-04-214-4855-1. https://doi.org/10.7916/D8XP72WF. eCollection 2014.
10. Alex Mohit A, Samii A, Slimp JC, Grady MS, Goodkin R. Mechanical failure of the electrode wire in deep brain stimulation. Parkinsonism Relat Disord. 2004;10:153–6.
11. Fernandez FS, Alvarez Vega MA, Antuna Ramos A, Fernandez Gonzalez F, Lozano Aragoneses B. Lead fractures in deep brain stimulation during long-term follow-up. Parkinsons Dis. 2010;2010:409356.
12. Yianni J, Nandi D, Shad A, Bain P, Gregory R, Aziz T. Increased risk of lead fracture and migration in dystonia compared with other movement disorders following deep brain stimulation. J Clin Neurosci. 2004;11:243–5.
13. Bayliss CE, Beanlands DS, Baird RJ. The pacemaker-twiddler's syndrome: a new complication of implantable transvenous pacemakers. Can Med Assoc J. 1968;99:371–3.
14. Astradsson A, Schweder PM, Joint C, Green AL, Aziz TZ. Twiddler's syndrome in a patient with a deep brain stimulation device for generalized dystonia. J Clin Neurosci. 2011;18:970–2.
15. Gelabert-Gonzalez M, Relova-Quinteiro J-L, Castro-García A. "Twiddler syndrome" in two patients with deep brain stimulation. Acta Neurochir. 2010;152:489–91.
16. Machado AG, Hiremath GK, Salazar F, Rezai AR. Fracture of subthalamic nucleus deep brain stimulation hardware as a result of compulsive manipulation: case report. Neurosurgery. 2005;57:E1318.
17. Sudhyadhom A, Haq IU, Foote KD, Okun MS, Bova FJ. A high resolution and high contrast MRI for differentiation of subcortical structures for DBS targeting: the Fast Gray Matter Acquisition T1 Inversion Recovery (FGATIR). Neuroimage. 2009;47(Suppl 2):T44–52.
18. Allert N, Schnitzler A, Sturm V, Maarouf M. Failure of long-term subthalamic nucleus stimulation corrected by additional pallidal stimulation in a patient with Parkinson's disease. J Neurol. 2012;259:1244–6.
19. Minafra B, Fasano A, Pozzi NG, Zangaglia R, Servello D, Pacchetti C. Eight-years failure of subthalamic stimulation rescued by globus pallidus implant. Brain Stimul. 2014;7:179–81.
20. Peppe A, Pierantozzi M, Bassi A, Altibrandi MG, Brusa L, Stefani A, et al. Stimulation of the subthalamic nucleus compared with the globus pallidus internus in patients with Parkinson disease. J Neurosurg. 2004;101:195–200.

Deep Brain Stimulation: Complications and Management

9

Steven Lange, Sameah Haider, Adolfo Ramirez-Zamora, and Julie G. Pilitsis

Introduction

Multiple studies have shown that deep brain stimulation (DBS) has been effective in reducing motor signs (tremor, bradykinesia, dystonia) and improving functionality and quality of life for patients with Parkinson's disease (PD). As DBS becomes more commonplace, maximizing perioperative safety is essential [19]. Although DBS is known to be a relatively safe and effective procedure, rates of complications in the literature vary because of categorical differences in their definition, the lack of large studies concerning surgical complications, underreporting of minor or common complications, and the difficulty in drawing precise comparisons across such studies. Also, a relatively small number of prospective studies have reported complications. Typically, these studies report a much higher rate of complications than retrospective studies [86]. Reporting of complications is usually reserved for atypical (and thus interesting) events. Though relatively rare as compared to other neurosurgical procedures, complications do occur. Wound infection (0–15% adverse event risk) and hardware complications (lead fracture, malposition, or migration) comprise the majority of long-term difficulties [9, 19]. The most severe complication is intracranial hemorrhage (ICH).

We conducted a literature review using PubMed and Google Scholar databases. Keywords used include "DBS," "complications," "adverse effects," "hardware," "biopsychosocial," and "mental health." Applicable sources were selected for retrieval with additional cross-reference search of cited literature. We grouped complications into the following classifications: (1) hardware-related, (2) biologic, (3) stimulation-related, and (4) cognitive-behavioral considerations. In addition, we offer means by which such complications can be avoided or addressed.

S. Lange · S. Haider · J. G. Pilitsis (✉)
Department of Neurosurgery, Albany Medical Center, Albany, NY, USA

A. Ramirez-Zamora
Department of Neurology, University of Florida, Gainesville, FL, USA

© Springer Nature Switzerland AG 2019
R. R. Goodman (ed.), *Surgery for Parkinson's Disease*,
https://doi.org/10.1007/978-3-319-23693-3_9

Surgical Complications

Serious surgical complications following DBS tend to be rare, such that a 30-day perioperative mortality and permanent neurological morbidity have been reported to be close to 0.4% and 1.0%, respectively, according to multicenter studies [72]. Other surgical complications include infection, hemorrhage, lead edema, venous infarction, confusion, pulmonary embolism, and peripheral nerve injury. Although a large number of patients experience an "adverse event" following DBS, most DBS-related air embolisms (AEs) are benign and transient [32].

Intracranial Complications

One of the most feared adverse events following DBS surgery is intracranial hemorrhage (ICH). Though it is most often asymptomatic, ICH can present symptomatically and lead to permanent neurological disability. The risk of symptomatic ICH causing permanent neurologic sequelae can be as high as 1.2%, while asymptomatic ICH may occur in as many as 3.4% of patients undergoing DBS for PD [18, 19, 60, 69, 80]. Ocular tilt, vertical diplopia from skew deviation, and vertical gaze palsy have been reported with midbrain hemorrhages, while subcortical ischemic strokes in the internal capsule and thalamus may present with hemiparesis, seizure, and mixed sensory findings. Though the etiology of ICH in DBS remains unclear, some hypothesized risk factors include the number of electrodes used for intraoperative microelectrode recording (MER), added force needed to pass the cannula through the cortex, trajectory through lateral ventricle, and use of microelectrodes with step-offs [51, 54, 69, 87]. ICH is most likely to occur with direct injury to vessels involved in the trajectory of electrode placement (Fig. 9.1). Additionally, DBS-associated insults have been linked to pre-existing vascular disease, small vessel vasospasm, edema, and mechanical irritation [80]. Furthermore, predisposing factors for ICH may include age, gender, perioperative hypertension, and use of anticoagulants [60, 69, 80]. It has been shown in at least one study that the rate of fatal ICH is much higher during electrode removal than implantation, and may be associated with more superficial hemorrhages. A review of 78 DBS electrodes removed at the Cleveland Clinic between October 2000 and May 2010 shows that 12.8% resulted in asymptomatic ICH, while 1300 leads implanted during the same period demonstrated a risk of asymptomatic hemorrhage of 2.0% per lead [40].

Direct trauma at the brain surface, injury to vessels in cortical sulci, or injury to deeper vascular structures (ependymal surface, choroid plexus) can increase the risk of ICH. Careful planning of placement and target trajectory should be made in order to avoid the ventricles and large veins, including thalamostriate veins and the highly vascularized choroid plexus in transventricular approaches. Planning of entry points, repeated verification of coordinates, and systematic monitoring of

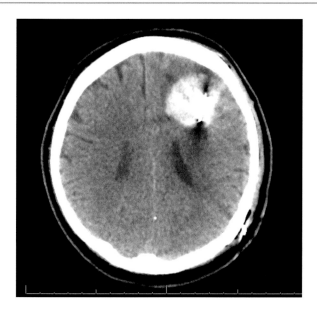

Fig. 9.1 A 56-year-old male who underwent ventral intermediate (Vim) thalamus DBS for essential tremor. On postoperative day three, he noted expressive aphasia. He was found to have this ICH. It resolved as did his symptoms with speech therapy after 6 months. He remains tremor free on the right side

systolic blood pressure are suggested in order to minimize the risk of peri- and postsurgical ICH [59]. Image-guided neuronavigation has been shown to reduce the severity of hemorrhage after DBS, effectively reducing the risk of ICH and aborted procedures [6, 41, 54]. The effect of DBS of the subthalamic nucleus (STN) on regional cerebral blood flow (rCBF) can be demonstrated by analyzing the changes in enhancement patterns using T1 double-dose gadolinium-enhanced brain magnetic resonance imaging (MRI). A decrease in contrast enhancement of ipsilateral small veins may suggest an alteration in venous blood flow around the electrode, though various studies of single-photon emission computerized tomography (SPECT) have also reported increases in regional cerebral blood flow (rCBF) during the first months of stimulation in subcortical structures, with correlation between rCBF and motor improvement [12, 62]. Treatment involves controlling blood pressure, stabilizing vital signs, maintaining euvolemia, avoiding hyperthermia, correcting coagulopathies, and mitigating seizure activity; resolution of symptoms is often witnessed in the postoperative period.

Venous infarction is another complication with the potential to evolve into delayed hemorrhage. Though a low incidence (<1.0%) has been reported in the literature, venous infarction can occur from transection or coagulation of large draining veins at the burr hole site [2, 59]. It has been suggested that more lateral burr hole placement, and placement away from surface veins as seen on MRI, likely decreases the risk of venous infarction. Unrecognized clinical sequelae, inconsistent follow-up imaging, comparability to microlesion effects, and variable correlation with vascular disease make venous infarction occasionally elusive; nevertheless, prolonged MER silencing arising while recording well-defined neuronal discharges can raise suspicion of potential infarction and may help the surgeon take precautionary measures to prevent adverse events. Although the actual mechanism of deep infarction is unknown, postulated theories include vasospasm from stimulation, lead compression of parenchyma, and microvascular vessel rupture [2]. It has been purported that ischemic strokes may be more common than previously thought, and have been more frequently associated with globus pallidus interna (Gpi)-DBS. Despite the severity for side effects reported, there is a wide variation in the incidence of hemorrhage and infarction in GPi-DBS [35]. Although STN-DBS was initially considered to be a more effective and reliable target than GPi-DBS leading to widespread use of STN DBS for the treatment of advanced stage PD, large, randomized trials have shown that STN and GPi DBS are similarly effective in improving motor function and quality of life at 36 months [75]. The rate of ICH is similar between the two targets [22]. Unilateral GPi-DBS may be favorable for patients who do not require bilateral surgery and who have more debilitating dyskinesia with small doses of medication, while STN DBS is currently heralded as the most promising intervention for young, highly levodopa-sensitive patients [22, 35, 47]. Infarction can be most readily avoided through a thorough understanding of a patient's preoperative status and likelihood of developing this postsurgical complication. Specifically, the use of high-resolution, contrast-enhanced T1-weighted MRI to delineate vascular anatomy and judicious stereotactic planning of lead trajectory has been proposed as a way of avoiding venous infarction; again, precautionary comprehensiveness and an orderly, well-managed operative regimen is likely to promote better outcomes in patients undergoing DBS for Parkinson's disease [46, 80].

Additionally, peri-electrode edema is another significant event that can result from DBS. Edema may occur in up to 6% of cases and cause focal neurological deficits, most commonly during the 96-hour postoperative window. In one study, cerebral edema—located near the tip, subcortical region and/or around the entire electrode—was noted at an average of 27 days after DBS surgery (range, 4–120 days). If symptomatic, symptoms resolve completely over an average of 33 days (range, 7–60), and include headache, focal neurologic deficits, and/or seizures. Though the nature and pathologic process remain undefined, studies have shown that the number of MER tracks correlate with the size and timing of edema [13]. The presence of edema in glial tissue is relevant to the short-term and long-term efficacy of the electrode and thus may impact acute and chronic adverse events [50]. Cranial MRI with specific settings can be used in patients with implanted hardware to identify vasogenic edema without a significant risk of imaging-related adverse events [85].

Systemic Complications

Because DBS surgery is often performed in a semi-sitting position with the cranial opening above the level of the heart, there is potential of venous air embolism (VAE) [10]. In actuality, however, this phenomenon remains rare. Air embolus, when it does occur, presents with acute-onset coughing, dyspnea, tachycardia, hypoxemia, and chest pain. Precordial Doppler is a safe, noninvasive monitor that can be used in the early detection of VAE in these procedures [28]. Venous complications (including venous infarction, as noted above) may be minimized by the administration of contrast during preoperative imaging so that burr hole locations may be placed remote to venous confluences or prominent surface veins, as disruption of venous vessels may predispose to VAE and venous infarction. Administration of 500 mL of normal saline to increase venous pressure at the beginning of surgery and minimized coughing may be beneficial prophylactic measures. If VAE does occur, bone wax to the diploë, copious irrigation of the field, and placement of the patient into a head-lowered position can avoid exacerbation of cardiopulmonary status [59]. If the patient remains hemodynamically unstable, the operation should be aborted, the patient placed in the lateral decubitus position with the right side up, and hemodynamic resuscitation undertaken.

The risk of seizures in DBS is low (0.2–2.3%), and is reportedly higher within the first 48 h after DBS surgery. Seizures are possibly one of the most underreported events, particularly if no intracranial complications arise concomitantly. Seizures are most likely to occur in the setting of ICH, peri-electrode edema, or ischemia, which increase the risk of postoperative seizures by 30- to 50-fold. A review of a consecutive series of DBS surgeries at a single institute showed that 7 (4.3%) of 161 cases who underwent 288 electrode implantations had generalized tonic-clonic seizures, and most (71%) only experienced a single seizure. Neither prophylaxis nor long-term treatment with anticonvulsants is recommended [56]. In a study of 233 patients diagnosed with PD, 56 surgical adverse events (SAE) occurred in 49 patients, 15 of which were seizures. Single tonic-clonic seizures were significantly related ($p = 0.002$) to ICH (cortical, thalamic, intraparenchymal, mesencephalic) and were reversible, with no signs of long-term clinical consequences [61]. It is reasonable to suspect that control of conditions which may precipitate ICH can help to modulate the incidence of seizures; avoidance of hemorrhagic risks and minimizing number of penetrations by electrodes is likely to reduce the incidence of DBS-related seizures. Postoperative computed tomography (CT) is critical to rule out ICH, since ICH is typically the most common reason for seizure occurrence especially during the first 12 h postimplantation. Close observation and monitoring of patients with a history of seizures may be warranted in the perioperative setting [29]. Despite the statistically significant relationship between ICH and seizure, MER and total amount of MERs do not significantly influence ICH or seizure incidence [61]. Anecdotally, the two seizures that have occurred

Summary for the Clinician

- Intracranial hemorrhage is a feared complication of unclear etiology that results from difficulties with electrode placement and may be affected by predisposing factors (age, gender, hypertension, anticoagulation) as well as direct injury to vascular structures.
- Suboptimal burr hole placement can increase the risk of venous infarction, which may be indicated by prolonged MER silencing.
- Peri-electrode edema causes focal neurologic deficits up to 2 months post-operatively and may predict long-term outcome.
- MRI is an effective method of delineating various surgical complications and improving patient outcomes.
- Venous air embolism is a rare complication that may be prevented with judicious burr hole placement, detected with precordial Doppler, and treated with bone wax to the diploe, copious irrigation of the field, and placement of patient into Trendelenberg position.
- DBS-related seizures are underreported events that occur in the setting of ICH, peri-electrode edema, ischemia, or revision surgery.
- Routine postoperative CT scanning is important for identifying ICH, since these are mostly asymptomatic, but raise the risk of seizures and may alter care.

in our series of several hundred patients were in patients who underwent revision surgery and were restarted on their original settings within 24 h postoperatively.

Hardware Complications

Hardware-related issues comprise a considerable percent of DBS-related complications. Various series have reported rates that range from 7% to 65%, though a better estimate of overall complications is approximately 8% per lead-year [30, 71]. Improved technologies and evolving surgical techniques, however, have limited hardware-related issues [33]. The emergent and expansive application of DBS to related conditions justifies greater focus on the probability and rate of surgical complications as they can be specific to subpopulation studied (Fig. 9.2). For instance, the rate of postoperative infection is higher in patients with Tourette's syndrome, possibly related to obsessive-compulsive traits associated with the disease. Simply stated, the more that procedures are performed (i.e., the greater the number of cases), the more complications there are, by virtue of the opportunity for mishap [5]. Appreciation of the various forms of device failure seen in DBS may aid clinicians in device implantation, complication identification, and avoidance of short-term and long-term complications.

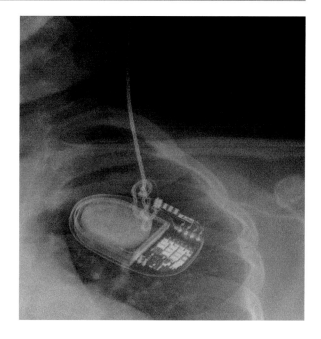

Fig. 9.2 A 38-year-old female with flipping of her generator showing evidence of curled extension at IPG site

An awareness of the outcomes of DBS surgery is likely to positively impact the quality of life of patients as well as reduce the morbidity associated with treatment and management.

Lead Migration

Hardware complications are defined as those events related to implanted leads (fracture or malposition/migration), the extension wire (erosion and fracture), or the IPG (malfunction, repositioning, or scar tissue growth, removal, or tightening) that required additional surgical intervention [41]. Postoperative imaging should be obtained following lead placement as a baseline to detect migration or misplacement [6]. Patients who experience suboptimal results often are found to have experienced lead migration. Although hardware-related complications are neither life-threatening nor concerning for permanent neurologic deficit, they do cause patient suffering and may pose a significant economic burden, especially considering their occurrence in approximately one-quarter of patients undergoing surgery for advanced PD [6, 16, 41]. Revision or explantation of hardware may double the total cost of care in addition to conferring added risk to the patient.

Lead migration (or, in some cases, misplacement) is the most frequent cause of hardware complication and surgical revision. DBS lead migration has been reported in 1.5–6.3% of patients, or ~4.4% of leads implanted, though these values may slightly vary depending on the specific institution and equipment used [2]. Lead migration can occur when the electrode has moved away from the optimal target, and is more likely to be a late development, though it may occur intraoperatively in the process of securing the DBS lead [2, 49]. When the electrodes shift from their original site of placement, the patient may experience: (1) a change in device efficacy, (2) acute changes in voltage requirements to sustain therapeutic benefits, (3) worsening of symptoms, and (4) other clinical manifestations that may include sudden severe change in cognition, mood, thoughts of suicide, seizure, and signs of stroke [49]. Dislocation of the lead may occur when the neurosurgeon attempts to secure the electrode, or when fixation of the lead to the skull is insufficient. Many surgeons use intraoperative fluoroscopy to image the lead before and after securement, especially when the clinical benefit is suboptimal [3, 16, 26]. The etiology of lead migration has also been attributed to patient-induced involuntary movement and improper location of the connector in the neck [2].

When there is a question of ineffective stimulation postoperatively, X-rays of the system should be obtained and impedances measured. A CT scan of the head with 1.5 mm cuts should also be obtained and lead location compared with the location in the postoperative period using fusion software. It needs to be recognized that as brain shift resolves, a slight change may occur in lead location relative to AC-PC over time and thus may not represent lead migration. Imaging studies have been able to isolate unpredictable movements in initially placed leads at any time between 6 months to 3 years after initial surgery when the patient notes decline in function, necessitating an immediate correction of lead placement [2, 16]. Fortunately, relocation of the lead restores therapeutic stimulation to the patient.

Issues with migration and fracture have spawned interest in improved lead securing devices and lower profile systems [30, 84]. Alternatively, some surgeons choose to use a titanium cranial plating system to secure the lead to the skull with good results [52]. When movement occurs, it is most common in the superior, rather than inferior, direction [77].

Lead Fracture

Lead fracture usually occurs at the burr hole anchorage site and depends upon the laxity of the mechanism adhering the electrode to the skull. Net forces acting upon the electrode can cause short-circuiting and actual physical disruption of the lead [9]. Repeated bending of the lead at a single point may also result in fracture, and lead fracture results in inadequate stimulation [6, 20, 59]. The incidence of lead fracture has been reported between 2.0% and 9.9% per patient, and may produce a short or open circuit in 0.9–9.9% of patients [2]. High rates of lead fracture have been correlated with placement of lead/extension connector in the upper neck or below the mastoid, and may be minimized by securing this connection on the calvarium [27]. The most important cause of lead fracture is rotational movement of the extension and the most common site is approximately 9–13 mm from the junction between the lead and extension cable [2, 20].

The mean time between DBS surgery and the diagnosis of lead fracture is 36 months, with a range of 7–84 months in one clinical study [20]. Excessive

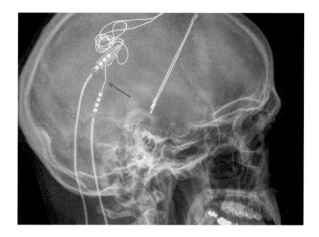

Fig. 9.3 A 38-year-old male with occupation in physical labor who noted shocking by his stimulator. Despite normal impedances and X-rays interpreted as negative, he was taken to the OR for exploration and found to have a gross break in his lead at the arrow site

tightening of the lead fixation plate is typically an immediate issue, though delayed fractures—potentially caused by changing the site of DBS lead/extension connection—may account for 5–10% of cases [30]. Lead fracture often can be circumvented by early intervention as well as a familiarity with the mechanism of choice. Additionally, the learning curve associated with implantation of DBS systems suggests that lead fracture can be better avoided by more experienced surgeons and seasoned technical acumen.

As in lead migration, X-ray, impedances, and CT should be obtained [41]. Component malfunction necessitates reoperation with removal and replacement of the damaged portion (Fig. 9.3). Strain-relief coils/loops may be helpful, especially in patients with dystonia or severe dyskinesias [59].

Infection

Infection remains the most common complication of DBS and may occur anywhere in the DBS system [5]. The most common pathogens are *Staphylococcus aureus* (most common), *Staphylococcus epidermidis*, and *Propionibacterium acnes* [4]. Risk factors for DBS-related infection include frontal subcutaneous connector placement, externalization of electrodes, and—in some literature—advanced age and immune compromise [4, 5].

Infections may be categorized as superficial incisional surgical site infection (SSI), deep incisional SSI, or organ/space SSI [4, 43]. There is a 4–12.2% risk of infection (mean of 5.6% in all performed procedures) per patient or 1.5–9.7% risk per lead, with most cases of infection occurring within the first 3 months postoperatively [2, 5]. The connector site tends to be the most common infection site, followed by the IPG pocket [9].

Many superficial infections can be treated with oral antibiotics, while deeper infections often require removal of the portion of the implanted hardware that is affected [59]. Infections require removal of the entire system, removal of a single component (lead, IPG, or extension), or only debridement, though partial hardware removal is often preferable and sufficient [2, 18]. Partial removal of hardware together with antibiotics should be attempted if the infected part is the IPG or extension wire, and if there is no evidence of infection over the brain lead, extensive cellulitis, or multiple drainage sites [5, 65]. Several studies indicate that infection by *S. aureus* should be treated with prompt local hardware removal and long-term antibiotic therapy, whereas other infections may be managed by an initial trial of antibiotics. Infections caused by *S. aureus* begin earlier, demonstrate classic signs of infection (e.g., purulence), and are less successfully treated with antibiotics or wound revision alone [5]. Nonetheless, early surgical treatment with partial hardware removal and appropriate antibiotic prophylaxis is considered in many cases to be effective conservative management for DBS-related infection, especially by *S. aureus* [4]. A study on the role of biofilm—a complex aggregate of microorganisms embedded in a self-produced polymeric matrix—in systemic infection and an awareness of biofilm formation can lead to higher success rates, less morbidity (pain, systemic upset, further surgical revision), and lower healthcare costs related to DBS-related infections [4, 64]. Reports of intracerebral infections are extremely rare after DBS [69]. Aseptic intracranial cyst development mimicking intracranial abscess is also a rare occurrence. This typically occurs months after implantation presenting with focal and worsening neurological symptoms [58]. Cultures and other signs of systemic inflammation are negative and treatment requires removal of hardware.

Avoidance of wound complication is best correlated with a consistent surgical team, strict enforcement of sterility, timeliness of the procedure, and use of prophylactic antibiotics perioperatively [18]. Prophylactic antibiotics are given before skin incision and redosed after 4–6 h. Additionally, it is advisable that all surgical personnel use double-gloving when hardware is on the field, that minimum personnel handle the hardware itself, and that care is taken to implant the hardware as soon as possible after package opening [59]. Certain surgical approaches that have been attempted to lower infection rates include: smaller incisions; meticulous surgical technique; shaving with clippers rather than razors; use of alcohol, betadine, and chlorhexidine skin prep; and copious irrigation of all wounds with bacitracin solution before closure [2, 4, 65].

Screening the nares of all patients for methicillin-sensitive *Staphylococcus aureus*/methicillin-resistant *Staphylococcus aureus* (MSSA/MRSA) prior to surgery may be beneficial in the prevention of nosocomial infection. Patients may be treated with mupirocin for 3 days prior to surgery as a prophylactic measure. Perioperative intranasal mupirocin also appears to decrease the incidence of surgical site infection when used as prophylaxis and is favorable for its low risk and low cost [31]. Irrigation of the operative field with bacitracin throughout the procedure and use of an intravenous cephalosporin and/or vancomycin perioperatively and for 23 h postoperatively can reduce the risk of DBS-related infection. The administration of vancomycin, however, should begin early in order to allow adequate time for tissue perfusion. Use of an oral antibiotic for up to 5 days postoperatively has also been shown to help prevent the incidence of infection, though not all medical centers routinely administer postoperative prophylaxis [2, 4]. Other common methods of limiting microbial infection include refraining from touching or coming in contact with the wound (due to bacterial colonization of the skin) and providing a barrier to the incision site. Preoperatively, a complete blood count (CBC) and urinalysis (UA) with culture and sensitivity may be ordered to rule out existing bacterial infection.

Prominence of the device under the scalp, neck, or subclavicular tissues predisposes to erosion through the skin. Surgical debridement, however, is crucial in the case of erosion without infection. In the event of erosion with negative cultures, management is at the surgeon's discretion [2, 25]. Placing permanent anchors only in deep tissue, and placing the IPG underneath muscle fascia rather than in subcutaneous fat, may also reduce the probability of erosion.

Summary for the Clinician
- Lead malposition/migration is the most frequent cause of hardware complication and surgical revision that may lead to change in efficacy, alteration of voltage requirements, worsening of symptoms, and neuropsychiatric sequelae.
- Lead fracture is caused by poor adherence to the skull, repeated bending, securement low on the calvarium, and rotational movement of the extension.
- X-ray and CT help to localize device changes that occur with lead migration and fracture.
- Checking impedances is important in identifying lead fractures.
- Infection of the DBS system is most often caused by *S. aureus* or *P. acnes* and may require oral antibiotics and/or hardware removal depending on the depth of infection.
- Attention to sterility, timeliness of the procedure, proper device placement, prophylactic antibiotics, and screening the nares for MSSA/MRSA may reduce the incidence of DBS-related infections.

Long-Term/Chronic Issues

Skin Complications

The incidence of skin erosion from both meta-analyses and case series ranges from 1% to 8.3%. In a retrospective study of 153 DBS implantations by a single implanter, the rate of skin erosion was 4.5% at a mean follow-up of 64 months [15]. The erosion of device components through the skin is often a subacute, or chronic, process; in a single center series of 85 patients from 2002 to 2009, 40% of skin complications occurred beyond 1-year postimplantation [66]. A retrospective series of 85 consecutive PD DBS patients in Germany suggested that age, hypertension, disease duration, and disease severity were not statistically significant risk factors for skin complications [66].

Patients should initially be counseled to avoid manipulation and excoriation of skin overlying device components: this includes avoidance of shaving one's scalp with direct blade-to-skin contact or even having a "military buzz cut" [69]. Upon noting evidence of skin erosion, the surgeon should be notified immediately and the wound assessed. Appropriate studies include blood cultures, device interrogation, and impedance checks. In the absence of local or systemic infection, device explantation may be avoided by reapproximating the wound, rerouting the hardware, and/or utilizing a well-vascularized scalp flap to protect exposed device components and repair the overlying skin defect. Lanotte and colleagues describe successful use of a rotational fasciocutaneous scalp flap supplied by branches of the superficial temporal artery [38].

A common site of skin erosion involves the extension lead at the connector site. Others describe a prophylactic measure to reduce the likelihood of skin erosion at the connector site; this method involves creating a recess within the calvarium to allow device components to sit flush and minimize overlying scalp tension [69]. If possible, one may also elect to cover the connector site with a portion of temporalis muscle. Any attempt to preserve device components should include local debridement and antibiotic washout.

Allergic reactions to DBS device components are faintly recognized in the literature; thus the true incidence of hypersensitivity responses cannot be extrapolated [48, 66]. If we draw from the body of literature surrounding spinal cord stimulation, we find that allergic reactions most commonly present as cutaneous manifestations overlying device components: these findings include erythema, pain, and pruritus in the absence of infectious stigmata [11]. If an allergic reaction is suspected, tissue culture and biopsy can both exclude infectious etiologies and confirm inflammatory infiltration. Additionally, cutaneous patch testing of antigens is often available through model-specific kits from the device manufacturer [68]. Of note, a negative yield from an allergy test kit has variable sensitivity and does not exclude the possibility. We have involved dermatology in these cases and ultimately have had to remove the device in one true allergy patient.

Loss of Efficacy

Common causes of poor efficacy include disease progression, improper patient selection, limited access to programming, lack of a multidisciplinary team, suboptimal lead location, and unrealistic patient expectations. In a single-center series of 728 patients, 29 patients (4%) presented with loss of motor improvement that was refractory to reprogramming and troubleshooting [19]. An earlier study of VIM DBS for essential tremor reported a loss of efficacy in 16% of patients (8 of 49) during a 40 month follow-up period [34]. The literature corroborates this finding; approximately 15–20% of VIM DBS patients report a loss of efficacy after an initial period of symptomatic improvement [55].

Current theories regarding loss of efficacy include stimulation tolerance, disease progression, and brain atrophy [19, 39, 44]. Observations of long-term DBS follow-up from several series describe the need for reduced programming thresholds to avoid unintended stimulation. Theoretically, as the brain atrophies, the volume of stimulation targets wanes, thus permitting stimulation current to spread beyond the intended nuclei [17, 44]. If stimulation tolerance were the predominant mechanism of loss of efficacy, we would expect increased programming thresholds at follow-up, which we sometimes do see [55]. In the realm of spinal cord stimulation, peri-electrode fibrosis has been implicated as a factor contributing to stimulation tolerance [37]. It is speculated that gliosis and inflammatory changes around the electrode tip insulate outbound stimulation, leading to rising impedances and ineffective stimulation over time. Neurohistological analysis from autopsies of long-term DBS patients demonstrates fibrillary gliosis and multinucleated giant cells, in concert with thin fibrous sheaths around electrode contacts [14, 67, 70]. Lastly, as diseases progress, DBS may no longer be able to provide meaningful benefit [7, 17].

In cases where patients have less effective stimulation, a Unified Parkinsons Disease Rating Scale (UPDRS) evaluation (on/off stimulation and on/off medication), device interrogation, and imaging studies should be obtained to expected stimulation benefit and confirm satisfactory lead location. A comparison of programming thresholds/impedances at each contact with prior stimulation requirements should be performed to better elucidate the cause of loss of efficacy [17, 44].

Reprogramming may offer significant benefit. Out of 50 patients presenting with long-term dissatisfaction with STN DBS, 22 patients reported amelioration of axial symptoms after reprogramming; this finding was observed even among patients presenting beyond 2 years postoperatively. The authors suspect that these symptoms were due to internal capsule stimulation [17]. Interleaved stimulation may be beneficial in refractory cases [57]. For a more detailed account of target-specific stimulation-related complications, please refer to the manuscript by Tong and colleagues [69].

When patients present with dissatisfaction from current therapy, it is advisable to assess the holistic well-being of the patient in a multidisciplinary fashion. Patients' expectations and hopes for surgery may not be met, despite appropriate preoperative counseling. In a series of 30 patients receiving STN DBS, 8 patients reported a subjective negative outcome of surgery at 3 months follow-up despite significant improvements in motor symptoms and quality of life [42]. All patients underwent accepted DBS screening protocols and preoperative approval independently by a movement disorder neurologist, neurosurgeon, psychiatrist, and a neuropsychologist. Not only should expectations be realistically addressed, but behavioral counseling and support should also remain an integral component of therapy as the disease progresses.

Summary for the Clinician
- The majority of potential complications declare themselves in the early postoperative period.
- Long-term complications are more likely to be related to hardware and efficacy.
- Skin erosion from underlying hardware components necessitates assessing the wound.
- While rare, the most at-risk location for skin erosion is the extension-connector interface.
- Loss of response to DBS may be due to a combination of disease progression and brain atrophy; this is supported by the need for reduced programming thresholds on long-term follow-up.
- Device interrogation and reprogramming is indicated with loss of efficacy.
- One must also assess the patient and caregivers' expectations, disposition, and outlook in a multidisciplinary fashion.

Stimulation-Related Considerations

Cognitive Changes

While DBS has been shown to improve motor symptoms of PD, it has also been associated with cognitive impairments at long-term follow-up. Patients with significant preoperative cognitive dysfunction are likely to have worse cognitive function postoperatively, thus emphasizing the importance of appropriate presurgical patient screening and neuropsychological assessment by clinical psychologists and psychiatrists [9]. It is thought that even moderate postsurgical cognitive impairment can shift patients with borderline impairment into the moderate-to-severe range of cognitive dysfunction, thus emphasizing the need for patient selectivity and prudent exclusion in questionable cases [79]. Experts agree that a critical element of favorable DBS outcomes is appropriate patient selection and preoperative evaluation. A multipronged approach to neuropsychological testing is valuable in establishing a reference point from which to compare future changes in cognitive, behavioral, and functional status [7, 21, 83]. Acceptable evaluation tools and functional subscales include the UPDRS, Mattis Dementia (MDRS) Rating Scale, Dementia Rating Scale (DRS), Stroop test (ST), Trail Making Test Part A and B (TMT A/B), Wisconsin Card Sorting Test (WCST), and the Parkinsons Disease Questionnaire (PDQ-39) [53, 78, 83]. While screening tools may be useful initially for patient selection and exclusion, they are not validated to detect more subtle changes in various cognitive domains [78].

At present, the neuromodulation community is still investigating the extent to which these changes are due to disease progression, surgery, and/or stimulation.

When evaluating the current literature, one should take note of the methodology used to assess cognitive function; cognitive screening tools are not designed to detect subtle changes in cognitive domains [78]. Additionally, studies commonly do not adjust for covariates as confounders when assessing overall cognitive function. Statistically significant differences between GPi and STN DBS on the MDRS and the Hopkins Verbal Learning Test have been reported [75]. Several recent studies have shown that declines in executive function seen postoperatively are transient and patients return to baseline by 6–12 months. Zangaglia and colleagues performed a prospective study evaluating cognitive function in 32 STN DBS patients and 33 medically managed PD patients. At 1 month postimplantation, the STN DBS group showed statistically significant declines in logical executive functioning and verbal fluency. Changes in the aforementioned cognitive variables returned to baseline by 12 months [83]. These findings were corroborated by two recent studies reporting transient declines in phonetic verbal fluency and frontal executive function that were recovered to preoperative baseline levels by 12 months after DBS implantation [81]. When compared to medically managed controls at 36 months follow-up, STN DBS patients showed impaired verbal fluency task scores. These findings suggest that declines in frontal executive function are transient while deteriorations in verbal fluency are more strongly associated with DBS stimulation. It is hypothesized that frontostriatal pathways involved in lexical retrial are disrupted by STN stimulation [83]. A meta-analysis of six randomized controlled trials also demonstrated a statistically significant decline in verbal fluency in DBS treated groups compared to medication-matched controls [53].

While STN DBS allows reductions in levodopa equivalent daily doses (LEDD), it has been noted that reductions in dopaminergic medication can contribute to worsening neuropsychiatric function [78]. Yamanaka and colleagues found a significant correlation between declining TMT A/B scores at 1 month and reduction in LEDD. The authors also remarked that the rate of LEDD reduction was more aggressive compared with medication reductions carried out in prior studies [81]. We recommend a gradual reduction in dopaminergic therapy after DBS implantation to avoid precipitating neurobehavioral signs of dopamine agonist withdrawal syndrome.

Neuropsychiatric Complications

Behavioral Changes

The synaptic connections found in the basal ganglia have implications on behavior due to their intimate relationships with limbic, subcortical, and prefrontal associative structures [82]. Noticeable changes in behavior after DBS implantation may be considered using two paradigms: exacerbation/mitigation of preexisting symptoms or new-onset psychiatric symptoms. If the behavioral changes are truly stimulation-related, the magnitude of change should be amenable to adjustments in stimulation parameters. Extrapolating the association between

DBS and long-term behavioral outcomes is more challenging due to the nature of underlying neurodegenerative disease.

Depression is a frequent comorbidity in those with neurodegenerative disorders. One of the greatest misfortunes in this patient population is the higher incidence of suicidality. Risk factors for attempted suicide include unmarried status, previous history of impulsivity, and postoperative depression [2, 69]. There is conflicting evidence regarding whether DBS is a risk factor for postoperative depression. A randomized prospective trial of DBS patients and wait-list controls did not establish any differences in the incidence of depression [74]. The incidence of suicide has been reported to range from 0.3% to 4.3% [32, 74]. In an international multi-center retrospective survey of more than 5000 patients with STN DBS, there was an increased risk of attempted and completed suicide rates in STN DBS patients in the first postoperative year, as compared with the lowest and the highest expected age-, gender-, and country-adjusted World Health Organization suicide rates (standardized mortality ratio). The single most important factor for a completed suicide was postoperative depression, whereas factors identified to be important for attempted suicide included a previous history of impulse control disorder, a previous history of suicide attempt, and a younger age of onset [73]. Analyzing the data of a large randomized Veterans Affairs (VA) study showed that suicidal ideation and behavior were similar in the DBS and best medication management cohorts when compared at 6 months postoperatively. The authors analyzed the DBS cohorts that underwent STN and GPi DBS, and found similar frequencies of suicidal ideations and behaviors. The author emphasizes the concern of developing suicidal behaviors associated with medication reduction postoperatively. Significant medical and psychiatric comorbidities, including the presence of pre- and postoperative depression, larger decreases in dopaminergic medications, and other general risk factors, may be associated with an increased risk for suicidal behavior after DBS surgery [76].

In order to appreciate behavioral changes from a clinical standpoint, one must establish the patient's preoperative baseline with extensive neuropsychological evaluation. This workup includes identification of risk factors concerning for poorer outcomes, such as: advanced age, disease stage, frontal lobe dysfunction, severe depression, or emotional instability [9, 21, 83]. Psychiatric disorders are not absolute contraindications to DBS treatment, granted the features of the disorder are not intrinsically disabling. Though psychiatric disorders and cognitive decline are among the greatest sources of disability in late-stage Parkinson's disease, they can also be influenced by the procedure itself [45]. The neuropsychiatric side effects of STN-DBS, in particular, include anxiety, apathy, decreased frontal cognitive function, decreased executive function, impulse control disorders, obsessive-compulsive disorder, and aggression. A systematic literature review on mood and behavioral changes after STN-DBS demonstrated that the most consistent side effect was decreased verbal fluency. Findings among a handful of studies regarding mood and affect were inconsistent and seldom clinically significant. Notable trends observed include: increase in depressive episodes, decrease in severity of depressive symptoms, increased apathy, and decreased anxiety [8].

Oftentimes caregivers and social support are the first to recognize changes in a patient's behavior; thus, it is appropriate to advise all stakeholders to be cognizant of behavior consistent with depression, mania, anxiety, apathy, or impulsivity. While the literature has suggested some associations between DBS target site and neuropsychiatric diatheses, individual presentations may vary; thus, it is safer to be alert to the gamut of possible behavioral changes. We recommend frequent follow-up in the early postoperative period in addition to an open letter of consultation to the patient's primary care physician describing what symptoms to be attuned to. The mental health provider in this multidisciplinary approach should have some experience with DBS patients and those with neurodegenerative disorders. Upon recognition of symptoms, the neurosurgeon or neurologist will begin a root-cause analysis to determine whether the observed behavioral changes are lead-location dependent, stimulation-related, or patient-related. For instance, Chan and colleagues describe three patients who presented with acute mania within the early postoperative follow-up. Imaging studies suggested that the lowest contact of the DBS lead was encroaching upon the substantia nigra. When stimulation was reassigned to a higher contact, the symptoms of mania gradually resolved over the ensuing weeks [9].

DBS safely improves motor control and quality of life in appropriately selected patients. The majority of affective changes observed postimplantation are amenable to reprogramming stimulation thresholds or instituting pharmacotherapy [69, 74, 82]. In vivo studies of STN DBS illustrated impaired serotonergic activity in the midbrain of rats in conjunction with depression-like behavior; these findings were accompanied by lower extracellular levels of serotonin per microdialysate analysis. Both serotonin levels and depression-like behavior were reversible with citalopram, a common selective serotonin reuptake inhibitor [33]. Thus, efforts to control symptoms with medication are reasonable in the absence of severely disabling behavioral changes. While we have largely limited our discussion to negative behavioral presentations in DBS patients, it is worth mentioning that many patients often display improvements in depression scores in long-term postoperative assessments [24]. While permanent long-term neuropsychological changes are uncommon, it is nonetheless important to maintain vigilance of their presentation.

Other Motor Symptoms

The presence of undesirable motor symptoms after DBS is largely a reversible phenomenon; patients, however, may choose to tolerate them for the benefit derived from DBS. These symptoms are due to propagation of electrical stimuli beyond the target tissue. Some adverse side effects tend to be idiosyncratic to the intended target site of stimulation. For instance, dysarthria and hypophonia have been reported after STN DBS, while dysarthria and ataxia are more common after GPi stimulation [23, 26, 69]. The breadth of stimulation-related motor symptoms includes dyskinesia, diplopia, dysarthria, dysphagia, and eyelid apraxia [63]. A wide variety of target-specific, stimulation-related side effects have been well described in prior reports [23, 69]. For the majority of patients, stimulation-related side effects are transient and amenable to reprogramming stimulation settings [1, 32]. Symptoms typically present in the early postoperative period (3–9 months), while both medication and stimulation settings are being optimized.

Summary for the Clinician
- Neuropsychiatric changes are common with progression of PD.
- Depression, anxiety, apathy, and psychosis rank among the most common symptoms. However, long-term assessments often depict improvements in mood and depression rating scales after DBS.
- There is no evidence to suggest a relationship between DBS and long-term behavioral changes. Permanent neuropsychological changes attributable to DBS are rare.
- Prior suicide attempt, or a history of impulse control problems, portends a higher risk for suicide attempt postoperatively.
- Extensive and ongoing neuropsychological evaluation remains a cornerstone of PD therapy.

Conclusion

DBS is a successful therapy for the treatment of PD and related movement disorders. Today, the STN and GPi are the most commonly used targets in PD. Acute and long-term results after DBS show a dramatic and stable improvement in a patient's clinical condition. Despite the array of surgical and hardware complications that have been reported following the procedure, serious postoperative complications are rare. Compared with medical therapy alone, DBS has been associated with a greater quality of life, including improvement in mobility, activities of daily living, and emotional well-being, and has not been shown to produce worse outcomes in those with greater preoperative disease severity. It is an attractive modality for patients who are refractory to pharmacologic treatment, and its efficacy depends on careful patient selection and efforts of a multidisciplinary team to reduce the incidence of complications and maximize benefit. The expanding use of DBS has necessitated a thorough understanding of optimal surgical techniques, many of which have been put forth by Baltuch and colleagues to address complication avoidance [36].

Summary for the Clinician
- DBS not only carries a lower risk of complications than lesional surgery but is also reversible.
- STN- and GPi-DBS have proven to be effective therapies for Parkinson's disease that are associated with a low incidence of serious postoperative complications and greater quality of life.
- DBS is an evolving surgical intervention that may benefit patients refractory to medical treatment.

References

1. Allert N, Markou M, Miskiewicz AA, Nolden L, Karbe H. Electrode dysfunction in patients with deep brain stimulation: a clinical retrospective study. Acta Neurochir. 2011;153:2342–9.
2. Bakay RAE, Smith AP. Deep brain stimulation: complications and attempts at avoiding them. Open Neurosurg J. 2011;4:42–52.
3. Baltuch GH, Stern MB. Deep brain stimulation for Parkinson's disease. Boca Raton: CRC; 2007.
4. Bhatia R, Dalton A, Richards M, Hopkins C, Aziz T, Nandi D. The incidence of deep brain stimulator hardware infection: the effect of change in antibiotic prophylaxis regimen and review of the literature. Br J Neurosurg. 2011;25(5):625–31.
5. Bjerknes S, Skogseid IM, Saehle T, Dietrichs E, Toft M. Surgical site infections after deep brain stimulation surgery: frequency, characteristics and management in a 10-year period. PLoS One. 2014;9(8):e105288.
6. Boviatsis EJ, Stavrinou LC, Themistocleous M, Kouyialis AT, Sakas DE. Surgical and hardware complications of deep brain stimulation. A seven-year experience and review of the literature. Acta Neurochir. 2010;152(12):2053–62.
7. Bronstein JM, Tagliati M, Alterman RL, Lozano AM, et al. Deep brain stimulation for Parkinson disease. Arch Neurol. 2011;68(2):165–71.
8. Castrioto A, Lhommee E, Moro E, Krack P. Mood and behavioural effects of subthalamic stimulation in Parkinson's disease. Lancet Neurol. 2014;13(3):287–305.
9. Chan DTM, Zhu XL, Yeung JHM, Mok VCT, et al. Complications of deep brain stimulation: a collective review. Asian J Surg. 2009;32(4):258–63.
10. Chang EF, Cheng JS, Richardson RM, Lee C, Starr PA, Larson PS. Incidence and management of air embolisms during awake deep brain stimulation in a large clinical series. Stereotact Funct Neurosurg. 2011;89(2):76–82.
11. Chaudhry ZA, Najib U, Jacobs WC, Sheikh J, Simopoulos TT. Detailed analysis of allergic cutaneous reactions to spinal cord stimulator devices. J Pain Research. 2013;6:617–23.
12. Choi BS, Kim YH, Jeon SR. Vascular changes caused by deep brain stimulation using double-dose gadolinium-enhanced brain MRI. Neural Regen Res. 2014;9(3):276–9.
13. Deogaonkar M, Nazzaro JM, Machado A, Rezai A. Transient, symptomatic, post-operative, non-infectious hypodensity around the deep brain stimulation (DBS) electrode. J Clin Neurosci. 2011;18(7):910–5.
14. DiLorenzo DJ, Danjovic J, Simpson RK, Takei H, Powell SZ. Neurohistopathological findings at the electrode-tissue Interface in long-term deep brain stimulation: systematic literature review, case report, and assessment of stimulation threshold safety. Neuromodulation. 2014;17:405–18.
15. Doshi PK. Long-term surgical and hardware-related complications of deep brain stimulation. Stereotact Funct Neurosurg. 2011;89:89–95.
16. Ellis TM, Foote KD, Fernandez HH, Sudhyadorm A, Rodriguez RL, Zeilman P, Jacobson CE, Okun MS. Reoperation for suboptimal outcomes after deep brain stimulation surgery. Neurosurgery. 2008;63(4):754–61.
17. Farris S, Giroux M. Retrospective review of factors leading to dissatisfaction with subthalamic nucleus deep brain stimulation during long-term management. Surg Neurol Int. 2013;4:69.
18. Fenoy AJ, Simpson RK. Management of device-related wound complications in deep brain stimulation surgery. J Neurosurg. 2012;116:1324–32.
19. Fenoy AJ, Simpson RK. Risks of common complications in deep brain stimulation surgery: management and avoidance. J Neurosurg. 2014;120(1):132–9.
20. Fernandez FS, Alvarez Vega MA, Antuna Ramos A, Fernandez Gonzalez F, Lozano AB. Lead fractures in deep brain stimulation during long-term follow-up. Parkinsons Dis. 2010; Article ID 409356, 4 pp.
21. Fields JA, Troster AI. Cognitive outcomes after deep brain stimulation for Parkinson's disease: a review of initial studies and recommendations for future research. Brain Cogn. 2000;42:268–93.

22. Follett KA, Weaver FM, Stern M, Hur K, et al. Pallidal versus subthalamic deep-brain stimulation for Parkinson's disease. N Engl J Med. 2010;362(22):2077–91.
23. Franzini A, Cordella R, Messina G, Marras CE, et al. Deep brain stimulation for movement disorders: considerations of 276 consecutive patients. J Neural Transm. 2011;118:1497–510.
24. Funkiewiez A, Ardouin C, Caputo E, Krack P, Fraix V, et al. Long term effects of bilateral subthalamic nucleus stimulation on cognitive function, mood, and behavior in Parkinson's disease. J Neurol Neurosurg Psychiatry. 2004;75:834–9.
25. Hariz MI. Complications of deep brain stimulation surgery. Mov Disord. 2002;17(3):S162–6.
26. Hariz MI. Deep brain stimulation: new techniques. Parkinsonism Relat Disord. 2014;20S1:S192–6.
27. Hariz MI, Johansson F. Hardware failure in parkinsonian patients with chronic subthalamic nucleus stimulation is a medical emergency. Mov Disord. 2001;16:166–8.
28. Hooper AK, Okun MS, Foote KD, Haq IU, et al. Venous air embolism in deep brain stimulation. Stereotact Funct Neurosurg. 2009;87(1):25–30.
29. Itakura T. Deep brain stimulation for neurological disorders: theoretical background. New York: Springer; 2015.
30. Joint C, Nandi D, Chir M, Parkin S, Gregory R, Aziz T. Hardware-related problems of deep brain stimulation. Mov Disord. 2002;17(3):S175–80.
31. Kallen AJ, Wilson CT, Larson RJ. Perioperative intranasal mupirocin for the prevention of surgical-site infections: systematic review of the literature and meta-analysis. Infect Control Hosp Epidemiol. 2005;26(12):916–22.
32. Kenney C, Simpson R, Hunter C, Ondo W, Almaguer M, Davidson A, Jankovic J. Short-term and long-term safety of deep brain stimulation in the treatment of movement disorders. J Neurosurg. 2007;106:621–5.
33. Kocabicak E, Yasin T. Deep brain stimulation of the subthalamic nucleus in Parkinson's disease: surgical technique, tips, tricks and complications. Clin Neurol Neurosurg. 2013;115(11):2318–23.
34. Koller WC, Lyons KE, Wilkinson SB, Troster AI, Pahwa R. Long-term safety and efficacy of unilateral deep brain stimulation of the thalamus in essential tremor. Mov Disord. 2011;16(3):464–8.
35. Krack P, Poepping M, Weinert D, Schrader B, Deuschl G. Thalamic, pallidal, or subthalamic surgery for Parkinson's disease? J Neurol. 2000;247(2):122–34.
36. Kramer DR, Halpern CH, Buonacore DL, McGill KR, et al. Best surgical practices: a stepwise approach to the University of Pennsylvania deep brain stimulation protocol. Neurosurg Focus. 2010;29(2):E3.
37. Kumar K, Toth C, Nath RK, Laing P. Epidural spinal cord stimulation for treatment of chronic pain – some predictors of success. A 15-year experience. Surg Neurol. 1998;50(2):110–20.
38. Lanotte M, Verna G, Panciani PP, Taveggia A, et al. Management of skin erosion following deep brain stimulation. Neurosurg Rev. 2009;32:111–5.
39. Larson PS. Deep brain stimulation for movement disorders. Neurotherapeutics. 2014;11(3):465–74.
40. Liu JK, Soliman H, Machado A, Deogaonkar M, Rezai AR. Intracranial hemorrhage after removal of deep brain stimulation electrodes. J Neurosurg. 2012;116(3):525–8.
41. Lyons KE, Wilkinson SB, Overman J, Pahwa R. Surgical and hardware complications of subthalamic stimulation: a series of 160 procedures. Neurology. 2004;63(4):612–6.
42. Maiser F, Lewis CJ, Horstkoetter N, Eggers C, Kalbe E, et al. Patients' expectations of deep brain stimulation, and subjective perceived outcome related to clinical measures in Parkinson's disease: a mixed-method approach. J Neurol Neurosrug Psychiatry. 2013;84:1273–81.
43. Mangram AJ, Horan TC, Pearson MI, Silver LC, Jarvis WR. Guideline for prevention of surgical site infection. Am J Infect Control. 1999;27:97–132.
44. Martinez-Ramirez D, Morishita T, Zeilman PR, Peng-Chen Z, Foote KD, et al. Atrophy and other potential factors affecting long term deep brain stimulation response: a case series. PLoS One. 2014;14(10):e111561.

ysis of hemorrhagic risk factors during deep brain

45. Mehanna R, Lai EC. Deep brain stimulation in Parkinson's disease. Transl Neurodegener. 2013;2:22.
46. Morishita T, Okun MS, Burdick A, Jacobson CE, Foote KD. Cerebral venous infarction: a potentially avoidable complication of deep brain stimulation surgery. Neuromodulation. 2013;16(5):407–13.
47. Obeso JA, Guridi J, Rodriguez-Oroz MC, Agid Y, et al. Deep-brain stimulation of the subthalamic nucleus or the pars interna of the globus pallidus in Parkinson's disease. N Engl J Med. 2001;345:956–63.
48. Oh MY, Abosch A, Kim SH, Lang AE, Lozano AM. Long-term hardware-related complications of deep brain stimulation. Neurosurgery. 2002;50(6):1268–76.
49. Okun MS, Zeilman PR. Parkinson's disease: guide to deep brain stimulation therapy: National Parkinson Foundation. Hagerstown, MD: 2014.
50. Paffi A, Camera F, Apollonio F, d'Inzeo G, Liberti M. Numerical characterization of intraoperative and chronic electrodes in deep brain stimulation. Front Comput Neurosci. 2015;9:2.
51. Park JH, Chung SJ, Lee CS, Jeon SR. Analysis of hemorrhagic risk factors during deep brain stimulation surgery for movement disorders: comparison of the circumferential paired and multiple electrode insertion methods. Acta Neurochir. 2011;153:1573–8.
52. Patel NV, Barrese J, DiTota RJ, Hargreaves EL. Deep brain stimulation lead fixation after Stimloc failure. J Clin Neurosci. 2012;19(12):1715–8.
53. Perestelo-Perez L, Rivero-Santana A, Perez-Ramos J, Serrano-Perez P, Panetta J, Hilarion P. Deep brain stimulation in Parkinson's disease: meta-analysis of randomized control trials. J Neurol. 2014;261:2051–60.
54. Piacentino M, Zambon G, Pilleri M, Bartolomei L. Comparison of the incidence of intracranial hemorrhage in two different planning techniques for stereotactic electrode placement in the deep brain stimulation. J Neurosurg Sci. 2013;57:63–7.
55. Pilitsis JG, Metman LV, Toleikis JR, Hughes LE, Sani SB, Bakay RAE. Factors involved in long-term efficacy of deep brain stimulation of the thalamus for essential tremor. J Neurosurg. 2008;109(4):640–6.
56. Pouratian N, Reames DL, Frysinger R, Elias WJ. Comhensive analysis of risk factors for seizures after deep brain stimulation surgery. J Neurosurg. 2011;115(2):310–5.
57. Ramirez-Zamora A, Kahn M, Campbell J, DeLaCruz P, Pilitsis JG. Interleaved programming of subthalamic deep brain stimulation to avoid adverse effects and preserve motor benefit in Parkinson's disease. J Neurol. 2015;262(3):578–84.
58. Ramirez-Zamora A, Levine D, Sommer DB, Dalfino J, Novak P, Pilitsis JG. Intraparenchymal cyst development after deep brain stimulator placement. Stereotact Funct Neurosurg. 2013;91(5):338–41.
59. Ranson M, Pope J, Deer T. Reducing risks and complications of interventional pain procedures. New York: Saunders; 2012.
60. Sansur CA, Frysinger RC, Pouratian N, Fu KM, Bittl M, Oskouian RJ, Laws ER, Elias WJ. Incidence of symptomatic hemorrhage after stereotactic electrode placement. J Neurosurg. 2007;107:998–1003.
61. Seijo F, Alvarez de Eulate Beramendi S, Santamarta Liebana E, Lozano Aragoneses B, Saiz Ayala A, Fernandez de Leon R, Alvarez Vega MA. Surgical adverse events of deep brain stimulation in the subthalamic nucleus of patients with Parkinson's disease: the learning curve and the pitfalls. Acta Neurochir. 2014;156:1505–12.
62. Sestini S, Ramat S, Formiconi AR, Ammannati F, Sorbi S, Pupi A. Brain networks underlying the clinical effects of long-term subthalamic stimulation for Parkinson's disease: a 4-year follow-up study with rCBF SPECT. J Nucl Med. 2005;46(9):1444–54.
63. Shipton EA. Movement disorders and neuromodulation. Neurol Res Int. 2012;2012. Article ID 309431. https://doi.org/10.1155/2012/309431.
64. Sievert DM, Ricks P, Edwards JR, Schneider A, Patel J. Antimicrobial-resistant pathogens associated with healthcare-associated infections: summary of data reported to the National Healthcare Safety Network at the Centers for Disease Control and Prevention, 2009-2010. Infect Control Hosp Epidemiol. 2013;34:1–14.

65. Sillay KA, Larson PS, Starr PA. Deep brain stimulation hardware-related infections: incidence and management in a large series. Neurosurgery. 2008;62:360–7.
66. Sixel-Doring F, Trenkwalder C, Kappus C, Hellwig D. Skin complications in deep brain stimulation for Parkinson's disease: frequency, time course, and risk factors. Acta Neurochir. 2010;152:195–200.
67. Sun DA, Yu H, Spooner J, Tatsas AD, Davis T, Abel TW, Kao C, Konrad PE. Postmortem analysis following 71 months of deep brain stimulation of the subthalamic nucleus for Parkinson disease. J Neurosurg. 2008;109(2):325–9.
68. Taverner MG. A case of an allergic reaction to a spinal cord stimulator: identification of the antigen with epicutaneous patch testing, allowing successful reimplantation. Neuromodulation. 2013;16:595–9.
69. Tong F, Ramirez-Zamora A, Gee L, Pilitsis J. Unusual complications of deep brain stimulation. Neurosurg Rev. 2014;38:245–52.
70. Vedam-Mai V, Yachnis A, Ullman M, Javedan SP, Okun MS. Postmortem observation of collagenous lead tip region fibrosis as a rare complication of DBS. Mov Disord. 2012;27(4):565–9.
71. Videnovic A, Metman LV. Deep brain stimulation for Parkinson's disease: prevalence of adverse events and need for standardized reporting. Mov Disord. 2008;23(3):343–9.
72. Voges J, Koulousakis A, Sturm V. Deep brain stimulation for Parkinson's disease. Acta Neurochir Suppl. 2007;97:171–84.
73. Voon V, Krack P, Lang AE, Lozano AM, Dujardin K, et al. A multicentre study on suicide outcomes following subthalamic stimulation for Parkinson's disease. Brain. 2008;131(10):2720–8.
74. Voon V, Kubu C, Krack P, Houeto JL, Troster AI. Deep brain stimulation: neuropsychological and neuropsychiatric issues. Mov Disord. 2006;21(14):S305–26.
75. Weaver FM, Follett KA, Stern M, Luo P, Harris CL, et al. Randomized trial for deep brain stimulation for Parkinson disease: thirty-six month outcomes. Neurology. 2012;79(1):55–65.
76. Weintraub D, Juda DE, Carlson K, Luo P, Sagher O, et al. Suicide ideation and behaviors after STN and GPi DBS surgery for Parkinson's disease: results from a randomised, controlled trial. J Neurol Neurosurg Psychiatry. 2013;84(10):1113–8.
77. Wharen RE, Putzke JD, Uitti RJ. Deep brain stimulation lead fixation: a comparative study of the Navigus and Medtronic burr hole fixation device. Clin Neurol Neurosurg. 2005;107(5):393–5.
78. Williams AE, Arzola GM, Strutt AM, Simpson R, Jankovic J, York MK. Cognitive outcome and reliable change indices two years following bilateral subthalamic nucleus deep brain stimulation. Parkinsonism Relat Diord. 2011;17(5):321–7.
79. Witt K, Daniels C, Reiff J, Krack P, et al. Neuropsychological and psychiatric changes after deep brain stimulation for Parkinson's disease: a randomised, multicentre study. Lancet Neurol. 2008;7:605–14.
80. Xiaowu H, Xiufeng J, Xiaoping Z, Bin H, Laixing W, Yiqun C, Jinchuan L, Aiquo J, Jianmin L. Risks of intracranial hemorrhage in patients with Parkinson's disease receiving deep brain stimulation and ablation. Parkinsonism Relat Diord. 2010;16(2):96–100.
81. Yamanaka T, Ishii F, Umemura A, Miyata M, Horiba M, et al. Temporary deterioration of executive function after subthalamic deep brain stimulation in Parkinson's disease. Clin Neurol Neurosurg. 2012;114:347–51.
82. York MK, Wilde EA, Simpson R, Jankovic J. Relationship between neuropsychological outcome and DBS surgery trajectory and electrode location. J Neuro Sci. 2009;287:159–71.
83. Zangaglia R, Pacchetti C, Pasotti C, Mancini F, Servello D, et al. Deep brain stimulation and cognitive functions in Parkinson's disease: a three-year controlled study. Mov Disord. 2009;24(11):1621–8.
84. Zibly Z, Sharma M, Shaw A, Yeremeyeva E, Deogaonkar M, Rezai A. Deep brain stimulation (DBS), lead migration, and the stimloc cap: complication avoidance. Neurol India. 2014;62(6):703–4.
85. Zrinzo L, Yoshida F, Hariz MI, Thornton J, Foltynie T, Yousry TA, Limousin P. Clinical safety of brain magnetic resonance imaging with implanted deep brain stimulation hardware: large case series and review of the literature. World Neurosurg. 2011;76(1–2):164–72.

86. Chin LS, Regine WF. Principles and practice of stereotactic radiosurgery. New York: Springer; 2015.
87. Alterman RL, Tagliati M. Deep brain stimulation for dystonia: patient selection, surgical technique, and programming. Open Neurosurg J. 2011;4(1-M2):29–35.

Part II

How Will DBS for PD Be Changing in the Near Future?

Closed-Loop Deep Brain Stimulation for Parkinson's Disease

10

R. Eitan, H. Bergman, and Z. Israel

Introduction

The advent of deep brain stimulation (DBS) as a therapeutic intervention has revolutionized the management of Parkinson's disease (PD) and several other neurological and psychiatric diseases. It is becoming increasingly obvious, however, that we may not be using this technology in a way that provides for optimal outcomes and/or maximum efficiency. Achieving such optimization might be assisted by a clear understanding of the mechanism of DBS action, the exact location of the stimulating electrodes, and the volume and structures activated by different stimulation settings, but to date such absolute clarity is still elusive. Surrogate biomarkers that reflect the clinical state have been sought and for some conditions have been found and validated. Automatic manipulation of DBS output in response to changes in these biomarkers may serve to improve clinical outcomes.

R. Eitan
Department of Medical Neurobiology (Physiology), Institute of Medical Research Israel-Canada (IMRIC), Edmond and Lily Safra Center (ELSC) for Brain Research, The Hebrew University, Jerusalem, Israel

H. Bergman
Department of Medical Neurobiology (Physiology), Institute of Medical Research Israel-Canada (IMRIC), Edmond and Lily Safra Center (ELSC) for Brain Research, The Hebrew University, Jerusalem, Israel

Department of Neurosurgery, Hadassah University Hospital, Jerusalem, Israel

Z. Israel (✉)
Department of Neurosurgery, Hadassah University Hospital, Jerusalem, Israel
e-mail: ISRAELZ@hadassah.org.il

© Springer Nature Switzerland AG 2019
R. R. Goodman (ed.), *Surgery for Parkinson's Disease*,
https://doi.org/10.1007/978-3-319-23693-3_10

Rationale

The activity of any individual constantly changes. For the patient with PD, functional status may additionally be influenced by ON-OFF motor fluctuations, dyskinesias, pain, dystonia, and emotional state that may or may not be associated with a drug regimen. However, contemporary DBS devices are "open loop" systems, *continuously* active with a constant unchanging output, irrespective of patient status. The efficiency of these DBS systems has been compared to the experience of driving a car with the cruise control locked in at high speed irrespective of the road or weather conditions [1]!

It has been suggested that a "closed-loop" or feedback control system wherein timing, intensity, and spatial and temporal pattern of stimulation are continuously titrated may have the potential to optimize outcome by improving efficacy, reducing side effects, limiting habituation, and decreasing the cost of treatment [2–5].

Feedback Loops

In its most basic form, a feedback system must include a sensor to monitor the status of the outcome. This information is then "fed back" into the implantable pulse generator (IPG) to adjust the output of the system to a preprogrammed optimum. Such endogenous feedback control is ubiquitous within many biological and technological systems. Some exogenous closed-loop systems that have been successfully developed include devices for the management of cardiac arrhythmias, epilepsy [6], and diabetes (Fig. 10.1).

Indeed, a contemporary view of the basal ganglia (BG) sees them functioning as a complex intrinsic feedback system, designed to optimize behavior [7]. This has been described as an "actor/critic" reinforcement or machine learning network [8]. When, however, "critic" function is lost, such as in the dopamine depleted Parkinsonian state, the BG lose the ability to detect state/action mismatch and to evaluate error in behavioral policy and the symptoms of PD ensue. Therapy of Parkinson's disease can be achieved by either dopamine replacement therapy or by modulation of the BG main axis "actor," as with DBS paradigms. DBS modulation

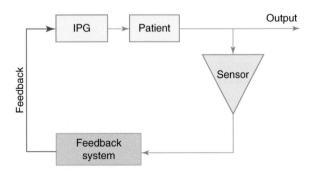

Fig. 10.1 Simplified concept of a closed-loop system. IPG implanted programmable generator

of the BG "actor" enables, by mechanisms as yet unknown, the restoration of close to normal state-to-action coupling.

DBS systems were developed with an "open-loop" design, with the *physician* intermittently intervening as both the sensor and feedback to "close the loop" by programming the implantable pulse generator (IPG) appropriately to the clinical condition of the patient. Although DBS surgery will often be very beneficial, there are obvious inherent issues with such a heuristic approach and an open-loop design. Programming may be extremely time consuming; patients may have to visit the clinic frequently in attempts to fine-tune their program; functional status between clinic visits is often suboptimal and the best program may never even be found!

Designing a Closed-Loop System

Crucial to a feedback system is the ability to both observe (*sense*) and control the current clinical status or surrogate biomarkers of that status. The surrogate biomarker or measurement should closely correlate with the clinical features of the disease. Interestingly, the ability to impose feedback control does not *necessarily* imply an understanding of the mechanisms by which a system works, which in the case of DBS is just as well, as these mechanisms are incompletely understood. The distinction has therefore recently been made between *phase responsive adaptive DBS (aDBS)*, designed to disrupt *causal* circuit dynamics, and *amplitude responsive aDBS*, wherein the magnitude of a surrogate biomarker signal determines the output [9]. The former implies knowledge of disease relevant circuit pathophysiology and how DBS works, and here greater insight may well enable us to change stimulation parameters to more efficiently manipulate pathological networks. In the latter, no direct understanding of underlying causal circuit dysfunction is implicit.

We consider that an optimal closed-loop DBS system should be able to sense and integrate information from multiple different sensitive and specific sources: (1) neural activity, (2) objective clinical signs (e.g., tremor, rigidity, bradykinesia, and posture/gait deficits), and (3) subjective clinical state (e.g., quality of life and activities of daily living). Appropriate integration of data from these various sources will inevitably rely on individualized algorithms based on population databases and machine learning predictions. These predictions should take into account a system of hierarchical control based on the *reliability* of the data source (1 > 2 > 3) and *temporal* features (e.g., 1 > 2 > 3 although this order may change) such that it is the most dependable, relevant, and most immediately available data that determines the stimulation paradigm with as little delay as possible. Other input to help fashion an individualized program may include predictive information from a population database, such as the dominant clinical features of disease (i.e., tremor vs. akinetic/rigid, the age of onset of disease, preoperative medication regimen, response to medication and genetic analysis, among others). Here we will review some of the progress that has been made toward developing elements of such a comprehensive system.

Neural Activity

Parkinson's disease research has contributed some very interesting clues toward our understanding of normal and pathological motor control. In the context of closed-loop or adaptive DBS, synchronous oscillations in the beta and gamma frequency have attracted most interest.

Desynchronized beta frequency oscillations are observed in many normally functioning cortico-basal ganglia networks [10, 11] and are thought to represent an idling rhythm, modulation of which is closely associated with the initiation and control of movement and behavior [12, 13]. Gamma frequency oscillations may also be important, normally playing a role at a relatively later stage of motor control, and encoding information related to limb *movement* rather than to muscle contraction initiation [14].

The description of an exaggerated pattern of synchronous beta frequency oscillatory firing in the subthalamic nucleus (STN) of the nonhuman primate 1-methyl-4-phenyl-1,2,3,6-tetrahydropyridine (MPTP) model [15] prompted the search for these pathophysiological features in the STN of human subjects with PD undergoing DBS surgery. Although there may be some significant differences between human PD and the primate MPTP model (notably in the peak frequency of oscillations in the beta band), the core features of increased neuronal firing rate [16], synchrony [17], and beta frequency oscillation [18] have all now been described in the dorsal/lateral (presumed somatosensory) part of the human Parkinsonian STN. We have been able to successfully exploit some of these electrical characteristics to assist in the automatic intraoperative identification and confirmation of surgical deep brain targets and their sub-territories [17, 19–23] (Fig. 10.2).

It is thought that this pathological excessive synchronous oscillation observed in motor networks in PD is normally prevented by active decorrelation of neurons in the network. However, in the dopamine depleted state the decorrelating mechanism is weakened or absent, possibly as a result of changes in the connectivity or strength of connections between or within BG nuclei [11, 24].

It has been proposed that the greatly enhanced beta synchronous oscillations observed in PD may limit the information coding capacity within the cortico-BG motor loops; novel processing is thereby impaired, favoring the status quo over new movement and giving rise to a bradykinetic state. In support of this idea, it has been observed that beta power is increased in PD patients who have their dopaminergic medication withdrawn [25]; beta power may correlate with PD symptom severity such as bradykinesia and rigidity [26–28] and beta power is suppressed by both levodopa and DBS *in proportion* to the clinical improvement they bring about [25, 29, 30]. Furthermore, surgically targeting structures that exhibit these pathophysiological hallmarks seem to determine optimal therapeutic outcome of DBS surgery [18]. In addition, there is accumulating evidence that part of the mechanism by which DBS works in PD may be by disrupting these pathological oscillations.

Exaggerated synchronous beta activity has been reported in many parts of the cortico-BG and BG-BG motor loops in PD, including the popular targets for DBS electrodes, such as the STN and the Globus Pallidus interna (GPi) and therefore

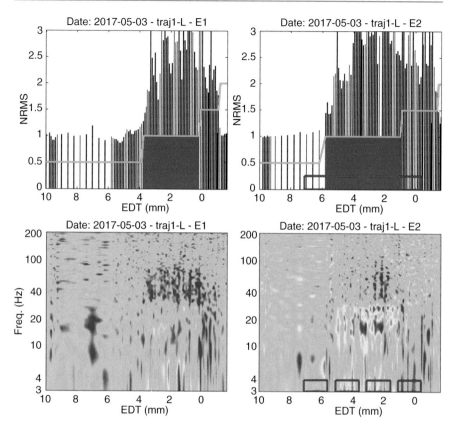

Fig. 10.2 Automatic microrecording in the STN. In the upper box, the normalized root mean square value of the MER signal (y-axis) is displayed as a function of the estimated distance to the target in the STN (x-axis). The green line overlay demonstrates the automatically detected entry into the STN, the transition from the oscillatory STN (red box overlay) to the nonoscillatory STN and the exit from the STN. In the lower box, the frequency spectrogram of oscillatory power (y-axis) is displayed as a function of the estimated distance to the target in the STN (x-axis). Both boxes show the proposed overlay of the contacts of the implanted permanent DBS electrode

may represent a good electrophysiological biomarker for a closed-loop paradigm in PD. It has recently been shown in both the primate MPTP model [31] and in human PD patients [32] that the distinguishing feature of pathological beta oscillations is most likely the longer duration of the oscillatory epochs. The amplitude of STN beta activity appears to increase in proportion to the burst duration, consistent with progressively increasing synchronization [33]. Targeting the longest oscillatory epochs in amplitude responsive closed-loop/adaptive paradigms has been highly successful [32, 34, 35]. Pathologically exaggerated synchronous oscillations in a narrow *gamma* frequency band have further been associated with the dyskinesias often seen in PD [36]. Oscillatory power in other frequency bands may also reflect the disease state/severity in various other diseases, such as theta frequency power in essential tremor [37] and alpha and theta frequency power in dystonia [26].

Although tempting, it is important however not to oversimplify, as normal motor control is far more complex than the simple interplay between oscillations in two frequency bands; oscillatory activity in one frequency band may not be a homogeneous function and rhythms of different frequencies may interact within the same signal to modulate different aspects of motor and non-motor activities.

Even on the assumption that beta activity is a sufficiently representative and reliable biomarker in PD, many questions remain. Which feature or features of the neural biomarker should we use (firing rate, pattern, other)? How should we be recording this data? Where is the optimal site to record the biomarker? And where should we stimulate for optimal results?

Choice of Neural Biomarker Feature

Both sampling algorithms and electrode characteristics will determine the type of data that can be recorded. In this respect, it is important to distinguish between local field potentials (LFPs) and spike data. LFPs are thought to represent the summation of all the extracellular subthreshold (synaptic and dendritic) activity and therefore reflect the global *input* into the sampled area. As a feedback signal, the LFP represents a population-based average metric. In contrast, neural spike data (single or multiunit activity) represents the cellular *output* of a structure [38]. Fortunately, there seems to be a correlative, predictive relationship between LFPs and spike activity [39–41].

The feature of the neural activity chosen as a biomarker for closed feedback is also closely related to the hardware that will be used to measure it. Microelectrodes, while excellent for acute recordings of spiking activity and LFPs (e.g., in the intraoperative setting), may not be appropriate for chronic recordings. Recording from single neurons demands a high sampling rate (optimally ≥ 10 kHz), is difficult to maintain over long periods of time and is subject to degradation due to the development of perielectrode gliosis. Furthermore, microelectrodes are unsuitable for stimulation due to current/density limitations that might result in tissue damage.

Macroelectrodes can be used to record LFPs, but not spiking activity, although we have recently shown that multiunit activity *can* be reliably recorded even from macro-contacts [42]. A practical sampling frequency for LFPs would be about 200 Hz, so high-frequency action potentials (300–5000 Hz) are filtered out, leaving only the slower (0.1–70 Hz) fluctuations. Thus, although the LFP signal is far more attractive in terms of computing power and memory, LFPs cannot be used to assess discharge rate. Monopolar LFP signals may be synchronized over long distances and may reflect volume conductance, such that closely spaced bipolar contacts within the target nucleus are more appropriate for focal recording [43].

LFPs have been demonstrated to reflect the patient's clinical state in PD and can be simultaneously recorded from the same deep brain electrode used for stimulation. LFPs also seem to stand the test of time, remaining consistent even many years after electrode implantation [44]. However, we still do not know the meaning of the total power of the LFP signal, which may be a function of electrode characteristics rather than physiological properties of the tissue or the patient. Despite these limitations, LFPs are considered to be an excellent candidate neural biomarker signal for the control of closed-loop DBS [45, 46].

Many aspects of such a system, using LFPs as a sensing modality and incorporating real-time automated closed-loop algorithms, have been successfully tested in an ovine epilepsy model analyzing hippocampal electrophysiology [46]. Similar promising results of LFP triggered closed-loop DBS have been reported in human PD patients in acute/short-term clinical experiments [34, 35].

Where Should We Record?

The optimal location to record may not necessarily be the best place to stimulate. A simple analogy to help understand this comes from the example of the thermostat, which may be best located at the center of a room, whereas the air conditioner might be better located on the ceiling or the heating system under the floor.

The primary motor cortex (M1) presents an attractive target for both recording and stimulation. Surgically, the M1 is easy to identify, very accessible and with relatively minimal and low risk intervention by way of either epidural [47] or subdural [48] electrodes. The classical box and arrow direct/indirect pathways model of the BG network suggests the M1 as the final common pathway of basal ganglia motor commands [49]. The same pathophysiological features of exaggerated synchronous beta oscillations have also been identified in the motor cortex [13]. However, studies of the effects of M1 stimulation on the clinical symptoms of PD have so far been largely disappointing, with no significant long-term improvement [50–56]. Progress in identifying the most appropriate cortical location to stimulate may improve this [57] and these efforts might be improved (or impaired) by cortical plasticity changes that may occur due to stimulation [58].

Recording from M1 on the other hand may provide very useful information for a closed-loop DBS paradigm. In our primate MPTP investigation, for example, M1 activity was successfully used to trigger GPi stimulation [59]. Several closed-loop paradigms were empirically explored, the most successful of which proved to be significantly more effective and more efficient than "standard" GPi stimulation. The empiric evolution of the optimal 80 ms delay (between cortical trigger and GPi stimulation) was most likely successful due to the 9–15 Hz frequency band of the primate MPTP model oscillations. Boraud viewed our approach as an attempt to restore cortical-BG connectivity, lost as part of the PD degenerative process [60].

This use of more than one implanted lead as a research tool has revealed aspects of the functional connectivity between structures and other useful disease relevant biomarkers. However, this is inherently more invasive, as it requires both a recording subdural cortical electrode and also a stimulating deep brain electrode. Individually, these both have an excellent safety profile [48].

The possibility of chronic cortical LFP recording with a subdural lead was demonstrated in a nonhuman primate [61] and the same group subsequently showed that not only was this also feasible and safe in human PD patients undergoing DBS surgery, but that the recorded electrocorticography (ECoG) signal could also be used for neurofeedback [36, 62].

Nevertheless, in order to minimize surgical intervention, most interest to date has been focused on recording from the same electrode that is surgically implanted for stimulation [34, 35, 63–65]. Data recorded from a stimulating lead, however, might be corrupted by stimulus artifacts, especially when high-frequency stimulation is used. The technology to enable simultaneous recording and stimulation has been a very challenging process of evolution [66–72], and in the setting of closed-loop DBS is probably best achieved by symmetric differential recording from contacts on the two adjacent sides of the stimulating contact [43, 70].

Where Should We Stimulate?

The debate concerning which of the two targets commonly implanted for PD (STN or GPi) might be clinically more beneficial is ongoing and unresolved despite several randomized prospective trials and multiple meta-analyses that have also included smaller nonrandomized trials [73–77]. One crucial issue often overlooked in these studies was validation of the location of the implanted electrode, which may have confounded outcome comparisons, but this debate is well beyond the scope of this chapter. There are, however, issues aside from those of clinical efficacy and potential side effects of trajectory and stimulation. The STN is both smaller and more cell dense than the GPi, thus a lead implanted in the STN may enable easier and more representative sampling of activity of the entire nucleus than a lead implanted in the GPi. By the same reasoning, stimulation of the STN might require less energy, and this is already borne out in clinical practice, with battery changes being more frequently necessary in patients implanted in the GPi. Furthermore, if indeed the stimulating electrode is to be used for recording too, LFP beta oscillations have been far better characterized for the Parkinsonian STN than for the GPi, at least in human PD patients, and caution should be exercised in extrapolating conclusions concerning STN beta to GPi beta. Finally, an electrode implanted in the STN could theoretically be extended, at least for recording, into the other BG output structure, the substantia nigra (SNr).

DBS of the Vim thalamic nucleus has been very successfully used for the amelioration of various forms of tremor, including PD tremor. Single unit recording has revealed very strong tremor-related activity in the Vim, the so-called tremor cells that seem to fire in bursts in tandem with the observed limb tremor. Early work showed that Vim cells exhibiting a large amount of power at tremor frequency were those best correlated with electromyography (EMG) activity during tremor, suggesting that some of these cells may have a causal role in the generation of tremor [37]. Alternatively, such tremor-related activity in the basal ganglia might be caused by proprioceptive feedback from the tremulous periphery. This dichotomy has not been resolved and has led us and others to assume that tremor may result from coupling of oscillators in different sites, both in the peripheral and central nervous systems [78, 79]. The optimal target for tremor control has also been debated for years and remains unresolved. Even highly successful initial control of tremor with well-positioned Vim DBS electrodes may be later compromised by accommodation and/or stimulation-induced complications, such as dysarthria and ataxia. Other targets that have been used with success include the caudal zona incerta and the posterior subthalamic area. The pioneering work of Coenen et al. in using diffusion-weighted magnetic resonance imaging to construct tractograms to assist DBS targeting [80] has highlighted the importance of including the dentato-rubro-thalamic tract in the stimulation volume for the control of tremor. This work represents a change of concept for DBS, away from targeting (and stimulating) nuclei and toward targeting and stimulating white matter tracts. This has important implications for closing the loop for tremor, as if the stimulating electrode is to be implanted in a tract rather than a nucleus, an alternative sensing solution must be contemplated, such as an appendicular subcutaneously implanted wireless tremor sensor.

Experience to Date

Attempts at clinical application of closed-loop DBS in humans have been concentrated within very few centers around the world. These are extremely challenging experiments to conduct and have therefore only been undertaken by groups who have a combined wealth of experience with DBS surgery and an established research track record in the pathophysiology of PD. Furthermore, most of the experience accumulated in humans has been in the acute postoperative phase with externalized electrode extensions and therefore have been time-limited to about 1 week for fear of infection and concern for patient comfort. The development of an implantable prototype DBS record/stimulate generator, the Activa PC + S by Medtronic may well change this.

1. Amplitude responsive adaptive DBS

    In two landmark studies, amplitude responsive aDBS was tested acutely in eight PD patients unilaterally [35] and subsequently bilaterally in four PD patients [34]. High-frequency DBS was activated only when the amplitude of beta in the STN exceeded a set threshold. The unilateral aDBS study demonstrated for the first time that not only was aDBS significantly more effective than continuous DBS (cDBS), but that stimulation on-time was also dramatically reduced. Random patterns of stimulation were ineffective. The bilateral study confirmed the significant reduction in stimulation on-time, but the effect on the motor Unified Parkinsons Disease Rating Scale (UPDRS) score (a reduction of 43%) was not compared with the clinical effect of cDBS. Amplitude responsive aDBS has also been tested in the nonhuman primate MPTP model with similar findings of at least equivalent clinical effect as cDBS and a 50% reduction in stimulation on-time [81].
    Reduced stimulation on-time has implications beyond saving battery energy. Less transfer of energy may also translate into fewer side effects, and this may explain the reduced dyskinesias [64, 65] and reduced speech side effects [63] observed with aDBS.

2. Coordinated reset stimulation

    DBS in its classical format may achieve desynchronization in the vicinity of the active electrode, but synchronization reappears within seconds of turning DBS off

[82]. On the premise that excessive pathological neuronal synchrony is a characteristic hallmark of PD [17], Tass et al. predicted that specifically counteracting abnormal neuronal synchrony with novel stimulation patterns might be clinically beneficial [83, 84] and might even obviate the necessity of time consuming individual programming. They coined the term "coordinated reset" (CR) to describe short "resetting" high-frequency pulse trains, directed through different electrode contacts at different times. In both primate models [85, 86] and in human PD studies [87] this technique has demonstrated not just acute improvement of motor function in response to stimulation, but also *persistent* effects even after cessation of stimulation.

This concept can also be harnessed in a closed-loop fashion, where synchrony is measured, preprocessed, and used as a feedback for the stimulation signal [88]. Stimulation could then be reduced or even stopped as soon as desynchronization is achieved. In practice, such a feedback signal is slow and might result in unsafe charge accumulation, although a technique to resolve this has recently been described [89, 90].

3. Temporally nonregular stimulation

Contemporary DBS systems utilize a regular temporal pattern of stimulation (i.e., the interval between each pulse does not vary as a function of time). *Random* patterns of stimulation, however, are ineffective [59]. Various patterns of temporally nonregular DBS have been found to be more effective at reducing bradykinesia (in a finger tapping task) than regular DBS [91]. These stimulation patterns were also more effective at suppressing beta band oscillatory activity in computational models. The same group has more recently used model-based computational evolution techniques to optimize the stimulation pattern [92]. This has not yet been utilized in a closed-loop format, although interestingly, the results of our own primate study had also shown that using cortical firing as a trigger resulted in a nonregular pattern of stimulation, which was also more effective than either standard or random DBS [59].

4. Phase amplitude decoupling

In humans, recording from the primary motor cortex during DBS surgery for PD using a subdural grid introduced via the same burr hole has revealed that in PD, STN spiking is *phase synchronized* with M1 LFPs in both lower frequency bands (4–30 Hz) and also with high-frequency activity over a broad spectral range (50–200 Hz) [93]. Furthermore, the *amplitude* of synchronized M1 gamma activity is itself rhythmically modulated by the *phase* of a lower-frequency rhythm, so-called phase-amplitude coupling (PAC), with the highest amplitude occurring at the *preferred* coupling phase such that "waves" of phase-synchronized cortical gamma activity precede the occurrence of STN spikes. In PD there is exaggerated PAC between STN β oscillations (measured with LFPs) and M1 γ oscillations (measured with ECoG) [94]. STN DBS has been shown to decrease PAC in the M1 [95], and therefore M1 PAC has been proposed as a potential feedback signal for closed-loop DBS [95, 96].

Beside the additional necessity for a cortical electrode in a system such as this, analyzing amplitude-phase coupling dynamics is computationally demanding. This same group has recently shown, in 3 PD patients, that a totally implanted system can use cortical signals for neurofeedback in real time [62]. The initial studies were performed in the acute perioperative phase, but more recently the same group has published their longer-term experience in 5 PD patients [97].

5. Fast Scan Cycling Voltammetry (FSCV)

Subsequent to their demonstration that STN DBS may involve the release of neurotransmitters [98, 99], the Mayo group led by Kendall Lee has developed implantable systems to measure parenchymal neurotransmitter concentrations, with the aim of using these as a closed feedback signal for DBS. In an evolving sequence of technological developments [100–102] with attractive acronyms (WINCS—Wireless Instantaneous Neurotransmitter Concentration Sensing [103], MINCS—Mayo Investigational Neuromodulation Control Systems [104]) they have shown proof-of-principle in the rodent [104, 105] and are working with larger animal models [106] and in humans [100] to demonstrate the utility of this approach.

6. Adaptive control using EMG and accelerometry

Two groups have tried to utilize tremor as a feedback symptom. Data from non-invasive surface electromyography [107] and accelerometry [108, 109] can be effectively integrated to both detect and even predict tremor. These algorithms have been successfully used in an adaptive ON-OFF DBS system to control tremor [109, 110]. Obvious limitations concern the subgroup of PD patients who have no or little tremor and that the onset of tremor may not be predictive of other features of PD.

Technological Advances

The field of DBS has witnessed some very significant technological advances, some of which may have direct relevance for the application of closed-loop paradigms.

Recently introduced into clinical use is the "segmented" electrode. Instead of continuously circumferential cylindrical contacts at the tip of the electrode, the contact can be "split" into several (three) parts, each of which can be programmed individually. Another prototype arranged up to 32 small contacts around the surface of the electrode. The conceptual purpose of these designs is to enable current steering and shaping of the stimulated volume in the event of a slightly malpositioned electrode. Current steering can be further augmented by combining an IPG with multiple independent current sources. Initial clinical experience has shown that even with "well positioned" electrodes, current steering can further improve the clinical benefit of DBS [111, 112]. This implies that there may be a particular sub-territory of the implanted nucleus that should be preferentially stimulated (and recorded from). Other studies recording LFPs from these contacts seem to support this idea [113, 114].

The advent of implantable rechargeable stimulators is significant inasmuch as closed-loop stimulation will inevitably be more power-hungry than classical stimulators, although there is still much to be desired in respect to battery size and technology.

The first closed-loop prototype sanctioned for clinical use is the Medtronic Activa PC + S which allows for LFP recording while simultaneously stimulating. This has recently been in groundbreaking clinical trials for various indications [97, 115] in several centers around the world. Although closed-loop technology is engineered into this device, it has not yet been authorized for routine clinical use.

Objective Clinical Signs

In terms of external input to a feedback system, elements of a *smart environment* could be utilized. The concept of an automated or smart home was first popularized in 1984 by the French journalist Bruno de Latour and possibly one of the first such homes to be built was described by the modern day visionary, Bill Gates around 1995 [116]. Smart homes have also become of increasing interest to the healthcare, communications, and security industries, among others. Healthcare elements that have already been realized include the ability to automatically detect if an elderly patient has fallen [117, 118], frailty status in the elderly [119], if a baby has stopped breathing, or if a cardiac patient has suddenly developed an arrhythmia. The concept of a smart *city* [120] has also now been added to our modern day technological lexicon even though it is not yet well defined. It is likely that next-generation high-speed broadband wireless networks (5G) may be configured to enable the inclusion of secured healthcare data.

What might be envisaged for the PD patient would be an individualized wireless home environment that can continuously monitor, for example, the patients' mobility [121], voice, and even facial expression. The patients' living space could be embedded with the necessary sensors including microphones, video cameras, and movement detectors [122]. Additional information, while outside the home environment, might come from accelerometers, gyroscopes, and magnetometers in a smartphone [123–125], or better still from a smart*watch* [126, 127], other wearable sensors [128–133], or even miniaturized implanted sensors.

Many sensors have been tested and validated for the assessment of tremor [130], bradykinesia [134, 135], gait [128, 135, 136], dysarthria, and dysphonia. Sensor-based programming for tremor and bradykinesia has been shown to be at least as good as clinician-based programming, or maybe even superior [137]. Rigidity assessment is more problematic as quantification is inherently subjective, however, one primate study did find good correlation using a system incorporating electromyographic recordings that detect and differentiate between active and actual resistance [138]. Two human studies have also addressed the issue of rigidity [139, 140].

To date, most research on *implantable* motion sensors has been performed on animals [141]; however, it is only a matter of time until such sensors can code for multiple measures [142] and be miniaturized sufficiently to justify subcutaneous implantation in humans. There may however be ethical issues to debate, as the type of information that continuous surveillance of this kind can provide is potentially open to abuse.

The PERFORM system is one such algorithm that has been validated to be able to fuse multiple parameters to remotely monitor the overall status of PD patients [143]. Such systems might even be utilized prior to a decision to operate [144], in order to assess and triage optimal patients for surgery and also intraoperatively [145]. Stored data might then be useful for programming the system subsequent to implantation.

Subjective Factors

When focusing on technology, we can sometimes get carried away and forget that our patients' subjective well-being should be at the center of our concern. Consider the occasional scenario of the neurologist, happy that his patient no longer has any objective signs of PD, but the patient simply does not feel right. A complete closed-loop system will have to provide for input of subjective information from the patient or his/her main supporter/caregiver. This might include data from questionnaires assessing activities of daily living (ADL), quality of life (QOL), or data from facial or voice recognition sensitive (and validated) for emotional and psychological state. This data could additionally be transferred and assessed telemetrically from long distance such that subjective patient status is continually monitored between visits. Most research to date exploring web-based telemetry or so-called eHealth programs has been in the field of cardiac failure, cardiac arrhythmias, hypertension, and diabetes. One study is exploring this modality to develop guidelines to help manage PD patients from afar [146].

The Future

Both the advocate and the skeptic would be well advised to take a deep breath; although we are not quite ready for full-scale implementation of closed-loop deep brain stimulation, most of the necessary technological elements are in advanced stages of development. This will happen, watch this space!

References

1. Modolo J, et al. Using "smart stimulators" to treat Parkinson's disease: re-engineering neurostimulation devices. Front Comput Neurosci. 2012;6:69.
2. Little S, Brown P. What brain signals are suitable for feedback control of deep brain stimulation in Parkinson's disease? Ann N Y Acad Sci. 2012;1265:9–24.

3. Hebb AO, et al. Creating the feedback loop: closed-loop neurostimulation. Neurosurg Clin N Am. 2014;25(1):187–204.
4. Priori A. Technology for deep brain stimulation at a gallop. Mov Disord. 2015;30(9):1206–12.
5. Beudel M, Brown P. Adaptive deep brain stimulation in Parkinson's disease. Parkinsonism Relat Disord. 2016;22(Suppl 1):S123–6.
6. Bergey GK, et al. Long-term treatment with responsive brain stimulation in adults with refractory partial seizures. Neurology. 2015;84(8):810–7.
7. Iskhakova L, Bergman H. Computational physiology of the basal ganglia, movement disorders and their therapy. In: Falup-Pecurariu C, et al., editors. Movement disorders curricula. Wien: Springer; 2017.
8. Schultz W, Dayan P, Montague PR. A neural substrate of prediction and reward. Science. 1997;275(5306):1593–9.
9. Meidahl AC, et al. Adaptive deep brain stimulation for movement disorders: the long road to clinical therapy. Mov Disord. 2017;32(6):810–9.
10. Khanna P, Carmena JM. Neural oscillations: beta band activity across motor networks. Curr Opin Neurobiol. 2015;32:60–7.
11. Wilson CJ. Oscillators and oscillations in the basal ganglia. Neuroscientist. 2015;21(5):530–9.
12. Cagnan H, Duff EP, Brown P. The relative phases of basal ganglia activities dynamically shape effective connectivity in Parkinson's disease. Brain. 2015;138(Pt 6):1667–78.
13. Heinrichs-Graham E, Wilson TW. Is an absolute level of cortical beta suppression required for proper movement? Magnetoencephalographic evidence from healthy aging. NeuroImage. 2016;134:514–21.
14. Muthukumaraswamy SD. Functional properties of human primary motor cortex gamma oscillations. J Neurophysiol. 2010;104(5):2873–85.
15. Bergman H, et al. The primate subthalamic nucleus. II. Neuronal activity in the MPTP model of parkinsonism. J Neurophysiol. 1994;72(2):507–20.
16. Deffains M, et al. Higher neuronal discharge rate in the motor area of the subthalamic nucleus of Parkinsonian patients. J Neurophysiol. 2014;112(6):1409–20.
17. Moshel S, et al. Subthalamic nucleus long-range synchronization-an independent hallmark of human Parkinson's disease. Front Syst Neurosci. 2013;7:79.
18. Zaidel A, et al. Subthalamic span of beta oscillations predicts deep brain stimulation efficacy for patients with Parkinson's disease. Brain. 2010;133(Pt 7):2007–21.
19. Zaidel A, et al. Delimiting subterritories of the human subthalamic nucleus by means of microelectrode recordings and a hidden Markov model. Mov Disord. 2009;24(12):1785–93.
20. Moran A, et al. Two types of neuronal oscillations in the subthalamic nucleus of Parkinson's disease patients. Mov Disord. 2008;23(1):S118.
21. Moran A, et al. Real-time refinement of subthalamic nucleus targeting using Bayesian decision-making on the root mean square measure. Mov Disord. 2006;21(9):1425–31.
22. Eitan R, et al. Asymmetric right/left encoding of emotions in the human subthalamic nucleus. Front Syst Neurosci. 2013;7:69.
23. Valsky D, et al. Stop! Border ahead: automatic detection of subthalamic exit during deep brain stimulation surgery. Mov Disord. 2017;32(1):70–9.
24. Canessa A, et al. Striatal dopaminergic innervation regulates subthalamic Beta-oscillations and cortical-subcortical coupling during movements: preliminary evidence in subjects with Parkinson's disease. Front Hum Neurosci. 2016;10:611.
25. Eusebio A, et al. Deep brain stimulation can suppress pathological synchronisation in Parkinsonian patients. J Neurol Neurosurg Psychiatry. 2011;82(5):569–73.
26. Kuhn AA, et al. Pathological synchronisation in the subthalamic nucleus of patients with Parkinson's disease relates to both bradykinesia and rigidity. Exp Neurol. 2009;215(2):380–7.
27. Neumann WJ, et al. Subthalamic synchronized oscillatory activity correlates with motor impairment in patients with Parkinson's disease. Mov Disord. 2016;31(11):1748–51.
28. Little S, et al. Beta band stability over time correlates with Parkinsonian rigidity and bradykinesia. Exp Neurol. 2012;236(2):383–8.

29. Kuhn AA, et al. Reduction in subthalamic 8-35 Hz oscillatory activity correlates with clinical improvement in Parkinson's disease. Eur J Neurosci. 2006;23(7):1956–60.
30. Little S, Brown P. Closed-loop programming: human perspective. In: Vitek J, editor. Deep brain stimulation: technology and applications. London: Future Medicine; 2014. p. 79–90.
31. Deffains M, Iskhakova L, Katabi S, Israel Z, Bergman H. Longer β oscillatory episodes reliably identify pathological subthalamic activity in Parkinsonism. Mov Disord. 2018.
32. Cagnan H, et al. Stimulating at the right time: phase-specific deep brain stimulation. Brain. 2016;140(1):132–45.
33. Tinkhauser G, et al. The modulatory effect of adaptive deep brain stimulation on beta bursts in Parkinson's disease. Brain. 2017;140(4):1053–67.
34. Little S, et al. Bilateral adaptive deep brain stimulation is effective in Parkinson's disease. J Neurol Neurosurg Psychiatry. 2016;87(7):717–21.
35. Little S, et al. Adaptive deep brain stimulation in advanced Parkinson disease. Ann Neurol. 2013;74(3):449–57.
36. Swann NC, et al. Gamma oscillations in the hyperkinetic state detected with chronic human brain recordings in Parkinson's disease. J Neurosci. 2016;36(24):6445–58.
37. Lenz FA, et al. Single unit analysis of the human ventral thalamic nuclear group: correlation of thalamic "tremor cells" with the 3-6 Hz component of Parkinsonian tremor. J Neurosci. 1988;8(3):754–64.
38. Buzsaki G, Anastassiou CA, Koch C. The origin of extracellular fields and currents--EEG, ECoG, LFP and spikes. Nat Rev Neurosci. 2012;13(6):407–20.
39. Michmizos KP, Sakas D, Nikita KS. Prediction of the timing and the rhythm of the Parkinsonian subthalamic nucleus neural spikes using the local field potentials. IEEE Trans Inf Technol Biomed. 2012;16(2):190–7.
40. Kuhn AA, et al. The relationship between local field potential and neuronal discharge in the subthalamic nucleus of patients with Parkinson's disease. Exp Neurol. 2005;194(1):212–20.
41. Weinberger M, et al. Beta oscillatory activity in the subthalamic nucleus and its relation to dopaminergic response in Parkinson's disease. J Neurophysiol. 2006;96(6):3248–56.
42. Winestone JS, et al. The use of macroelectrodes in recording cellular spiking activity. J Neurosci Methods. 2012;206(1):34–9.
43. Marmor O, et al. Local vs. volume conductance activity of field potentials in the human subthalamic nucleus. J Neurophysiol. 2017; https://doi.org/10.1152/jn.00756.2016.
44. Giannicola G, et al. Subthalamic local field potentials after seven-year deep brain stimulation in Parkinson's disease. Exp Neurol. 2012;237(2):312–7.
45. Priori A, et al. Adaptive deep brain stimulation (aDBS) controlled by local field potential oscillations. Exp Neurol. 2013;245:77–86.
46. Afshar P, et al. A translational platform for prototyping closed-loop neuromodulation systems. Front Neural Circuits. 2012;6:117.
47. Rasche D, Tronnier VM. Clinical significance of invasive motor cortex stimulation for trigeminal facial neuropathic pain syndromes. Neurosurgery. 2016;79(5):655–66.
48. Panov F, et al. Intraoperative electrocorticography for physiological research in movement disorders: principles and experience in 200 cases. J Neurosurg. 2016;126(1):122–31.
49. Albin RL, Young AB, Penney JB. The functional anatomy of basal ganglia disorders. Trends Neurosci. 1989;12(10):366–75.
50. Cilia R, et al. Extradural motor cortex stimulation in Parkinson's disease. Mov Disord. 2007;22(1):111–4.
51. De Rose M, et al. Motor cortex stimulation in Parkinson's disease. Neurol Res Int. 2012;2012:502096.
52. Lefaucheur JP. Treatment of Parkinson's disease by cortical stimulation. Expert Rev Neurother. 2009;9(12):1755–71.
53. Munno D, et al. Neuropsychologic assessment of patients with advanced Parkinson disease submitted to extradural motor cortex stimulation. Cogn Behav Neurol. 2007;20(1):1–6.
54. Zwartjes DG, et al. Motor cortex stimulation for Parkinson's disease: a modelling study. J Neural Eng. 2012;9(5):056005.

55. Bentivoglio AR, et al. Unilateral extradural motor cortex stimulation is safe and improves Parkinson disease at 1 year. Neurosurgery. 2012;71(4):815–25.
56. Moro E, et al. Unilateral subdural motor cortex stimulation improves essential tremor but not Parkinson's disease. Brain. 2011;134(Pt 7):2096–105.
57. Kern K. et al. Detecting a cortical fingerprint of Parkinson's disease for closed-loop neuromodulation. Front Neurosci. 2016;10(110).
58. Boakye M. Implications of neuroplasticity for neurosurgeons. Surg Neurol. 2009;71(1):5–10.
59. Rosin B, et al. Closed-loop deep brain stimulation is superior in ameliorating parkinsonism. Neuron. 2011;72(2):370–84.
60. Boraud T. Closed-loop stimulation: the future of surgical therapy of brain disorders? Mov Disord. 2012;27(2):200.
61. Ryapolova-Webb E, et al. Chronic cortical and electromyographic recordings from a fully implantable device: preclinical experience in a nonhuman primate. J Neural Eng. 2014;11(1):016009.
62. Khanna P, et al. Neurofeedback control in Parkinsonian patients using electrocortigraphy signals accessed wirelessly with a chronic, fully implanted device. IEEE Trans Neural Syst Rehabil Eng. 2016;25(10):1715–24.
63. Little S, et al. Adaptive deep brain stimulation for Parkinson's disease demonstrates reduced speech side effects compared to conventional stimulation in the acute setting. J Neurol Neurosurg Psychiatry. 2016;87(12):1388–9.
64. Rosa M, et al. Adaptive deep brain stimulation in a freely moving Parkinsonian patient. Mov Disord. 2015;30(7):1003–5.
65. Rosa M, et al. Adaptive deep brain stimulation controls levodopa-induced side effects in Parkinsonian patients. Mov Disord. 2017;32:628.
66. Campbell GA, Crawford IL. A gated electronic switch for stimulation and recording with a single electrode. Brain Res Bull. 1980;5(4):485–6.
67. Ferrer AZ, Fernández-Guardiola A, Solís H. Electronic circuit breaker for recording and stimulation from same electrode. Electroencephalogr Clin Neurophysiol. 1978;45(2):299–301.
68. Hatzopoulos A, Theophilidis G. A simple electronic unit allowing extracellular recording and stimulation through the same wire hook or suction electrode. J Neurosci Methods. 1984;11(3):169–72.
69. Rossi L, et al. An electronic device for artefact suppression in human local field potential recordings during deep brain stimulation. J Neural Eng. 2007;4(2):96–106.
70. Stanslaski S, et al. Design and validation of a fully implantable, chronic, closed-loop neuromodulation device with concurrent sensing and stimulation. IEEE Trans Neural Syst Rehabil Eng. 2012;20(4):410–21.
71. Al-ani T, et al. Automatic removal of high-amplitude stimulus artefact from neuronal signal recorded in the subthalamic nucleus. J Neurosci Methods. 2011;198(1):135–46.
72. Harding GW. A method for eliminating the stimulus artifact from digital recordings of the direct cortical response. Comput Biomed Res. 1991;24(2):183–95.
73. Williams NR, Foote KD, Okun MS. STN vs. GPi deep brain stimulation: translating the rematch into clinical practice. Mov Disord Clin Pract. 2014;1(1):24–35.
74. Odekerken VJ, et al. GPi vs STN deep brain stimulation for Parkinson disease: three-year follow-up. Neurology. 2016;86(8):755–61.
75. Odekerken VJ, et al. Subthalamic nucleus versus globus pallidus bilateral deep brain stimulation for advanced Parkinson's disease (NSTAPS study): a randomised controlled trial. Lancet Neurol. 2013;12(1):37–44.
76. Weaver FM, et al. Randomized trial of deep brain stimulation for Parkinson disease: thirty-six-month outcomes. Neurology. 2012;79(1):55–65.
77. Okun MS, Foote KD. Subthalamic nucleus vs globus pallidus interna deep brain stimulation: the rematch: will pallidal deep brain stimulation make a triumphant return? Arch Neurol. 2005;62(4):533–6.
78. Arkadir D, et al. In quest of the oscillator(s) in tremor: are we getting closer? Brain. 2014;137(Pt 12):3102–3.

79. Lee RG, Stein RB. Resetting of tremor by mechanical perturbations: a comparison of essential tremor and Parkinsonian tremor. Ann Neurol. 1981;10(6):523–31.
80. Coenen VA, et al. One-pass deep brain stimulation of dentato-rubro-thalamic tract and subthalamic nucleus for tremor-dominant or equivalent type Parkinson's disease. Acta Neurochir. 2016;158(4):773–81.
81. Johnson LA, et al. Closed-loop deep brain stimulation effects on Parkinsonian motor symptoms in a non-human primate – is Beta enough? Brain Stimul. 2016;9(6):892–6.
82. Meissner W, et al. Subthalamic high frequency stimulation resets subthalamic firing and reduces abnormal oscillations. Brain. 2005;128(Pt 10):2372–82.
83. Tass PA. A model of desynchronizing deep brain stimulation with a demand-controlled coordinated reset of neural subpopulations. Biol Cybern. 2003;89(2):81–8.
84. Tass PA. Phase resetting in medicine and biology: stochastic modelling and data analysis. Berlin: Springer; 1999.
85. Tass PA, et al. Coordinated reset has sustained aftereffects in Parkinsonian monkeys. Ann Neurol. 2012;72(5):816–20.
86. Wang J, et al. Coordinated reset deep brain stimulation of subthalamic nucleus produces long-lasting, dose-dependent motor improvements in the 1-methyl-4-phenyl-1,2,3,6-tetrahydropyridine non-human primate model of parkinsonism. Brain Stimul. 2016;9(4):609–17.
87. Adamchic I, et al. Coordinated reset neuromodulation for Parkinson's disease: proof-of-concept study. Mov Disord. 2014;29(13):1679–84.
88. Montaseri G, et al. Synchrony suppression in ensembles of coupled oscillators via adaptive vanishing feedback. Chaos. 2013;23(3):033122.
89. Popovych OV, et al. Pulsatile desynchronizing delayed feedback for closed-loop deep brain stimulation. PLoS One. 2017;12(3):e0173363.
90. Popovych OV, Lysyansky B, Tass PA. Closed-loop deep brain stimulation by pulsatile delayed feedback with increased gap between pulse phases. Sci Rep. 2017;7(1):1033.
91. Brocker DT, et al. Improved efficacy of temporally non-regular deep brain stimulation in Parkinson's disease. Exp Neurol. 2013;239:60–7.
92. Brocker DT, et al. Optimized temporal pattern of brain stimulation designed by computational evolution. Sci Transl Med. 2017;9(371).
93. Shimamoto SA, et al. Subthalamic nucleus neurons are synchronized to primary motor cortex local field potentials in Parkinson's disease. J Neurosci. 2013;33(17):7220–33.
94. de Hemptinne C, et al. Exaggerated phase-amplitude coupling in the primary motor cortex in Parkinson disease. Proc Natl Acad Sci U S A. 2013;110(12):4780–5.
95. de Hemptinne C, et al. Therapeutic deep brain stimulation reduces cortical phase-amplitude coupling in Parkinson's disease. Nat Neurosci. 2015;18(5):779–86.
96. Gunduz A, et al. Proceedings of the second annual deep brain stimulation think tank: what's in the pipeline. Int J Neurosci. 2015;125(7):475–85.
97. Swann NC, et al. Chronic multisite brain recordings from a totally implantable bidirectional neural interface: experience in 5 patients with Parkinson's disease. J Neurosurg. 2017;128(2):605–16.
98. Lee KH, et al. Neurotransmitter release from high-frequency stimulation of the subthalamic nucleus. J Neurosurg. 2004;101(3):511–7.
99. Shon YM, et al. High frequency stimulation of the subthalamic nucleus evokes striatal dopamine release in a large animal model of human DBS neurosurgery. Neurosci Lett. 2010;475(3):136–40.
100. Bennet KE, et al. A diamond-based electrode for detection of neurochemicals in the human brain. Front Hum Neurosci. 2016;10:102.
101. Jang DP, et al. Paired pulse voltammetry for differentiating complex analytes. Analyst. 2012;137(6):1428–35.
102. Koehne JE, et al. Carbon nanofiber electrode array for electrochemical detection of dopamine using fast scan cyclic voltammetry. Analyst. 2011;136(9):1802–5.

103. Chang SY, et al. Wireless fast-scan cyclic voltammetry measurement of histamine using WINCS--a proof-of-principle study. Analyst. 2012;137(9):2158–65.
104. Chang SY, et al. Development of the Mayo investigational neuromodulation control system: toward a closed-loop electrochemical feedback system for deep brain stimulation. J Neurosurg. 2013;119(6):1556–65.
105. Grahn PJ, et al. A neurochemical closed-loop controller for deep brain stimulation: toward individualized smart neuromodulation therapies. Front Neurosci. 2014;8:169.
106. Min HK, et al. Dopamine release in the nonhuman primate caudate and putamen depends upon site of stimulation in the subthalamic nucleus. J Neurosci. 2016;36(22):6022–9.
107. Graupe D, et al. Adaptively controlling deep brain stimulation in essential tremor patient via surface electromyography. Neurol Res. 2010;32(9):899–904.
108. Shukla P, et al. A neural network-based design of an on-off adaptive control for deep brain stimulation in movement disorders. Conf Proc IEEE Eng Med Biol Soc. 2012;2012:4140–3.
109. Malekmohammadi M, et al. Kinematic adaptive deep brain stimulation for resting tremor in Parkinson's disease. Mov Disord. 2016;31(3):426–8.
110. Khobragade N, Graupe D, Tuninetti D. Towards fully automated closed-loop deep brain stimulation in Parkinson's disease patients: a LAMSTAR-based tremor predictor. Conf Proc IEEE Eng Med Biol Soc. 2015;2015:2616–9.
111. Contarino MF, et al. Directional steering: a novel approach to deep brain stimulation. Neurology. 2014;83(13):1163–9.
112. Pollo C, et al. Directional deep brain stimulation: an intraoperative double-blind pilot study. Brain. 2014;137(7):2015–26.
113. Bour LJ, et al. Directional recording of subthalamic spectral power densities in Parkinson's disease and the effect of steering deep brain stimulation. Brain Stimul. 2015;8(4):730–41.
114. Fernández-García C, et al. Directional local field potential recordings for symptom-specific optimization of deep brain stimulation. Mov Disord. 2017;32:626.
115. Vansteensel MJ, et al. Fully implanted brain-computer interface in a locked-in patient with ALS. N Engl J Med. 2016;375(21):2060–6.
116. Gates B. The road ahead. London: Penguin Books; 1995.
117. Palmerini L, et al. A wavelet-based approach to fall detection. Sensors (Basel). 2015;15(5):11575–86.
118. Wu F, et al. Development of a wearable-sensor-based fall detection system. Int J Telemed Appl. 2015;2015:576364.
119. Schwenk M, et al. Wearable sensor-based in-home assessment of gait, balance, and physical activity for discrimination of frailty status: baseline results of the Arizona frailty cohort study. Gerontology. 2015;61(3):258–67.
120. Wikipedia. Smart City. Available from: https://en.wikipedia.org/wiki/Smart_city.
121. Jalal A, Kamal S, Kim D. A depth video sensor-based life-logging human activity recognition system for elderly care in smart indoor environments. Sensors (Basel). 2014;14(7):11735–59.
122. Siddiqi MH, et al. Video-based human activity recognition using multilevel wavelet decomposition and stepwise linear discriminant analysis. Sensors (Basel). 2014;14(4):6370–92.
123. Kostikis N, et al. Smartphone-based evaluation of Parkinsonian hand tremor: quantitative measurements vs clinical assessment scores. Conf Proc IEEE Eng Med Biol Soc. 2014;2014:906–9.
124. Parviainen J, et al. Adaptive activity and environment recognition for mobile phones. Sensors (Basel). 2014;14(11):20753–78.
125. Shoaib M, et al. Fusion of smartphone motion sensors for physical activity recognition. Sensors (Basel). 2014;14(6):10146–76.
126. Garcia-Ceja E, et al. Long-term activity recognition from wristwatch accelerometer data. Sensors (Basel). 2014;14(12):22500–24.
127. Wile DJ, Ranawaya R, Kiss ZH. Smart watch accelerometry for analysis and diagnosis of tremor. J Neurosci Methods. 2014;230:1–4.

128. Buchman AS, et al. Associations between quantitative mobility measures derived from components of conventional mobility testing and Parkinsonian gait in older adults. PLoS One. 2014;9(1):e86262.
129. Cancela J, et al. Wearability assessment of a wearable system for Parkinson's disease remote monitoring based on a body area network of sensors. Sensors (Basel). 2014;14(9):17235–55.
130. Heldman DA, et al. Clinician versus machine: reliability and responsiveness of motor endpoints in Parkinson's disease. Parkinsonism Relat Disord. 2014;20(6):590–5.
131. Mera T, et al. Kinematic optimization of deep brain stimulation across multiple motor symptoms in Parkinson's disease. J Neurosci Methods. 2011;198(2):280–6.
132. Mera TO, et al. Feasibility of home-based automated Parkinson's disease motor assessment. J Neurosci Methods. 2012;203(1):152–6.
133. Sanchez-Ferro A, Maetzler W. Advances in sensor and wearable technologies for Parkinson's disease. Mov Disord. 2016;31(9):1257.
134. Campos-Romo A, et al. Quantitative evaluation of MPTP-treated nonhuman Parkinsonian primates in the HALLWAY task. J Neurosci Methods. 2009;177(2):361–8.
135. Chien SL, et al. The efficacy of quantitative gait analysis by the GAITRite system in evaluation of Parkinsonian bradykinesia. Parkinsonism Relat Disord. 2006;12(7):438–42.
136. Hubble RP, et al. Wearable sensor use for assessing standing balance and walking stability in people with Parkinson's disease: a systematic review. PLoS One. 2015;10(4):e0123705.
137. Pulliam CL, et al. Motion sensor strategies for automated optimization of deep brain stimulation in Parkinson's disease. Parkinsonism Relat Disord. 2015;21(4):378–82.
138. Mera TO, et al. Objective quantification of arm rigidity in MPTP-treated primates. J Neurosci Methods. 2009;177(1):20–9.
139. Endo T, et al. A novel method for systematic analysis of rigidity in Parkinson's disease. Mov Disord. 2009;24(15):2218–24.
140. Prochazka A, et al. Measurement of rigidity in Parkinson's disease. Mov Disord. 1997;12(1):24–32.
141. Baker JJ, et al. Continuous detection and decoding of dexterous finger flexions with implantable myoelectric sensors. IEEE Trans Neural Syst Rehabil Eng. 2010;18(4):424–32.
142. Li Y, et al. A low power, parallel wearable multi-sensor system for human activity evaluation. Proc IEEE Annu Northeast Bioeng Conf. 2015; 2015.
143. Tzallas AT, et al. PERFORM: a system for monitoring, assessment and management of patients with Parkinson's disease. Sensors (Basel). 2014;14(11):21329–57.
144. Lieber B, et al. Motion sensors to assess and monitor medical and surgical management of Parkinson disease. World Neurosurg. 2015;84(2):561–6.
145. Papapetropoulos S, et al. Objective monitoring of tremor and bradykinesia during DBS surgery for Parkinson disease. Neurology. 2008;70(15):1244–9.
146. Marceglia S, et al. Web-based telemonitoring and delivery of caregiver support for patients with Parkinson disease after deep brain stimulation: protocol. JMIR Res Protoc. 2015;4(1):e30.

Is There a Role for MRI-Guided Focused Ultrasound Lesioning for PD?

11

Carter S. Gerard and Ryder Gwinn

Summary of Key Points
- Surgical intervention has had a role in the treatment of Parkinson's disease during the last 80 years.
- Focused ultrasound was first developed in the 1950s, but has had a renaissance in the last decade due to improved technology such as phased array transducers and MR-thermography.
- Focused ultrasound allows for accurate lesioning with real-time lesion quantification and constant neurological monitoring.
- Multiple reports have described the use of focused ultrasound in neuro-oncology, movement disorders, psychiatric disorders, and pain syndromes.
- Focused ultrasound was recently approved in the United States for unilateral thalamotomy for essential tremor.
- Multiple trials are currently underway for use of focused ultrasound for the treatment of Parkinson's disease.

Introduction

Transcranial magnetic resonance imaging (MRI)-guided focused ultrasound (MRgFUS) is a potent technology for the treatment of intracranial pathologies. The use of focused ultrasound for the treatment of Parkinson's disease (PD) was first described over 70 years ago. However, long treatment times and the need for a

C. S. Gerard · R. Gwinn (✉)
Department of Neurosurgery, Swedish Neuroscience Institute, Seattle, WA, USA
e-mail: Ryder.gwinn@Swedish.org

© Springer Nature Switzerland AG 2019
R. R. Goodman (ed.), *Surgery for Parkinson's Disease*,
https://doi.org/10.1007/978-3-319-23693-3_11

craniotomy resulted in limited clinical use in favor of other forms of stereotactic lesioning. The development of additional technologies during the last two decades has produced a renaissance for focused ultrasound in the treatment of intracranial pathologies. Advances in MRI now allow for real-time quantification of the lesion and improved targeting. Improvements in ultrasound phased array technologies are now able to negotiate varying skull thicknesses obviating the need for a craniotomy. MRgFUS currently grants the ability to create accurate lesions, without an incision, with immediate effect and real-time neurologic monitoring, qualities that have special appeal to the functional neurosurgeon. Ongoing clinical trials for MRgFUS include treatment of stroke, tumor, pain, psychiatric disorders, and movement disorders. In this chapter, we will discuss the current literature, technical considerations, and clinical trials of MRgFUS in the treatment of Parkinson's disease.

History

The study of acoustics was first described over 4000 years with the first application in medicine only occurring in the last century [1]. In the 1930s, Karl Theadore Dussik, a neurologist at the University of Vienna, would be the first to use ultrasound in the field of medicine in an unsuccessful attempt to visualize brain tumors. In the 1940s, the surgeon John Julian reported the use of ultrasound to diagnose abdominal disease such as ileus and bowel obstruction. He went on to describe the use of ultrasound to diagnose breast cancer and the intraoperative localization of a brain tumor after a craniotomy was performed. The 1950s would see further applications including the use of ultrasound for detection of ovarian lesions and for the documentation of fetal growth as reported by Dr. Ian Donald at the University of Glasgow [2]. Around the same time, Hertz and Elder described the use of ultrasound to evaluate mitral valve disease and thereby introduced echocardiography to the world [3].

The destructive potential of ultrasonography had been recognized in 1915 while developing SONAR, yet further investigation to develop a lesioning tool for medical treatment would not be published for another 40 years [4]. While working at Columbia University in 1944, John G Lynn and Tracy J. Putnam published their findings on the effects of high-intensity focused ultrasound (HIFU) on the brain. They described limited parenchymal lesions and inadvertently causing skin necrosis. Histological evaluation of the lesions showed ganglion cells to be most sensitive to damage, followed by glial cells, and very little effect on blood vessels [2]. In the early 1950s, Dr. Thomas Ballentine, a neurosurgeon, and Padmaker Lele, a neurophysiologist, working at Massachusetts General Hospital were able to use focused ultrasound to target the Edinger–Westphal nucleus and cause reversible pupillary dilatation in cats. The group also commented on the wide threshold which made it difficult to predict when a permanent lesion would occur [1]. During this same period, William and Francis Fry, physicists at the University of Illinois, were studying the ability to cause discreet lesions in the CNS with HIFU (Fig. 11.1a) [5, 6]. The Fry brothers would later partner with a neurosurgeon,

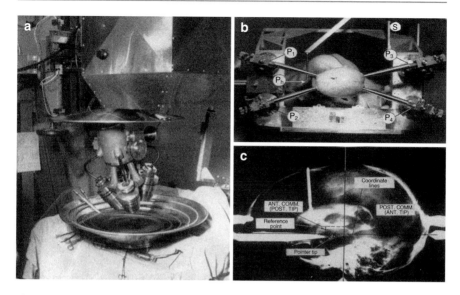

Fig. 11.1 The first human trial of high-intensity focused ultrasound (HIFU) was performed with a device with four sound transducers developed by William Fry at the University of Illinois (**a**). The patient's head was immobilized (**b**) and ventriculography was then performed to facilitate targeting (**c**). Treatments were time consuming and could last up to 14 h

Russell Myers, at the University of Iowa for clinical trials. In 1958, they published a series of 54 patients with Parkinson's disease who were treated with focused ultrasound to lesion the substantia nigra and ansa lenticularis. The principal steps of the procedure were numerous and included ventriculography, target acquisition, craniotomy, dural opening, and ablation (Fig. 11.1b, c). Treatments were time consuming lasting greater than 10 h [7]. During the following decades, multiple notable neurosurgeons, including Lars Leksell, Peter Lindstrom, and John Jane Sr., continued to study the properties and investigate the use of HIFU in the field of neurosurgery.

The technology was aggressively trialed in the 1980s in ophthalmology and gynecology. However, HIFU failed to gain significant clinical application in the field of neurosurgery due to lack of real-time imaging during ablations and the need for craniotomy due to beam distortion from bone. These limitations would finally be overcome in the 1990s with the development of phased arrays of ultrasound transducers [8] and the incorporation of MRI with MR thermography [9]. By incorporating multiple phased array transducer elements, a computed tomography (CT) scan could be used to calculate the amount of energy required at each array to overcome the irregularities of the skull. The incorporation of MRI, with MRI thermography, allowed for accurate targeting and real-time quantification of the lesions [8]. MRI-guided focused ultrasound has become an expanding area of basic and clinical research. MRI-guided focused ultrasound has been involved in multiple human clinical trials including obsessive-compulsive disorder [10], essential tremor [11–13], neuropathic pain [4, 14], and Parkinson's disease [15–17].

Fig. 11.2 Modern focused ultrasound (FUS) systems (Exblate 4000 by InSightec) now consist of up to 1024 element phased array transducers arranged within a hemispheric helmet (Fig. 11.2)

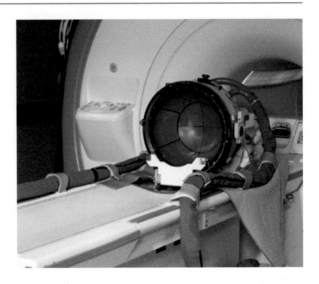

Core Concepts of MRI-Guided Focused Ultrasound

Modern FUS systems (Exblate 4000 by InSightec) now consist of up to 1024 element phased array transducers arranged within a hemispheric helmet (Fig. 11.2). Phase correction now allows for each transducer to be modified in order to mitigate interference from the skull [18]. Similar to the multibeam arrangement used in stereotactic radiosurgery, the sound waves then intersect at the center of the hemisphere and reach a high intensity capable of creating a distinct lesion [19].

Thermal lesions are caused by absorption of ultrasonic energy by the target tissue. This allows for temperature elevation in tissue sufficient to cause tissue denaturing and coagulation in seconds [20]. Nonthermal damage is thought to be caused by cavitation. Cavitation occurs when sounds waves cause liquids to become a gas. If the acoustic waves continue, the bubbles can cause damage to surrounding tissues and should therefore be avoided when a precise lesion is required [20].

Confirmation of the focal site of maximal beam intensity is critical due to the importance of anatomic accuracy. MRI thermography is able to detect the temperature at target and throughout the brain. Real-time temperature measurement ensures sufficient energy is absorbed for ablation and that remote sites are unaffected.

Treatment Protocol for Functional Procedure with MRI-Guided Focused Ultrasound

In addition to the appropriate disease-specific work-up and counseling, all patients must undergo an MRI and CT scan of the brain in order to be considered for treatment. Clinical trials have shown that a small subset of patients with thick craniums showed poor outcomes due to insufficient ultrasonic penetration of the skull.

Therefore, the CT scan of the skull is now reviewed prior to the day of treatment to determine if the patient is a candidate for MRI-guided FUS.

After informed consent is obtained, the patient presents to the preoperative area where a single peripheral IV is placed. The patient's head is shaved and a stereotactic frame is placed with local anesthetic. A rubber skirt with a central aperture is then fitted around the patient's head, ensuring that it is as low as possible. This is typically worn in a "head band" position. The patient is then placed supine on the MRI table while the stereotactic frame is fixed to the base plate of the MRI transducer (Fig. 11.3a). The transducer helmet is then positioned so that the center of the hemisphere is at the target zone. The elastic membrane allows for a water tight seal and the area above the skirt is later filled with water. This ensures that the scalp is cooled throughout the procedure.

MR images are then obtained, in addition to a tracking scan that registers the transducer location to the MRI. The transducer helmets can then be readjusted to ensure that the target is at the center of the hemispheric helmet. The CT images are then fused to the MRI. The information from the CT allows the system to adjust the output of each transducer in relation to the shape and thickness of the skull, intracranial calcification, and areas of air (such as the paranasal sinuses). Markers are placed on the images at the border of the ventricles to assist in movement detection.

Once the target is determined, the treatment plan is assessed to ensure that at least 700 of the 1024 elements of the transducer are active and that the skull area involved is at least 250 cm². These requirements ensure that the energy is sufficiently disseminated over the skull. The target is initially treated with

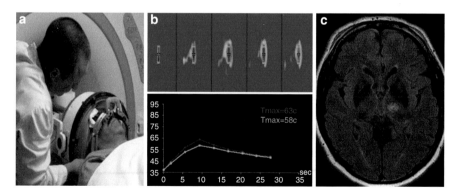

Fig. 11.3 After the patient is placed in a stereotactic frame, he or she is fixed into the transducer array on the magnetic resonance imaging (MRI) table (**a**). Once planning is complete, the target is treated with subtherapeutic sonications. This produces heating from 40 to 45 °C. The test allows for confirmation that the area of temperature increase is at the intended target. Any targeting errors are corrected and the sonications are slowly lengthened to increase the target temperature. A target temperature of 51–55 °C may produce reversible clinical effects. A lesion is then created by delivering sonications that reach temperatures of 55–60 °C. MRI thermography allows for real-time monitoring of target temperatures (**b**). Post-operative MRI Flair sequence shows a left VIM lesion (**c**)

subtherapeutic sonications. This produces heating from 40 to 45 °C. This test allows for confirmation that the area of temperature increase is at the intended target. Any targeting errors are corrected and the sonications are slowly lengthened to increase the target temperature. A target temperature of 51–55 °C will produce reversible clinical effects. A lesion is then created by delivering sonications that reach temperatures of 55–60 °C (Fig. 11.3b, c). Patients are assessed after each sonication for both efficacy and side effects. When the treatment is completed, the frame is removed and the patient is taken to recovery. A unilateral thalamotomy typically lasts 3–4 h [18]. Patients are monitored in the hospital overnight and discharged home the following day.

Is There a Role for MRI–Guided Focused Ultrasound Lesioning for PD?

Prior to the use of dopamine, lesioning of the GPi and thalamus were mainstays for the treatment of Parkinson's disease [21, 22]. While lesioning continued for refractory cases of PD, the success of subthalamic nucleus (STN) and globus pallidus internus (GPI) deep brain stimulation (DBS) even further decreased the practice. The development of MRI-guided FUS and the appeal of incisionless surgery have renewed interest in lesioning for PD.

Magara et al. [16] published the first clinical series for the treatment of PD with MRI-guided FUS in 2014. The authors reported a series of medically refractory patients who had a pallidothalamic tractotomy performed. The ExAblate Neuro device (InSightec, Tirat Carmel, Israel) was used at the following coordinates: ×7.5 mm lateral to mid-commissural point, y at the mid-commissural point, and z at the mid-commissural point. The initial four patients received a single sonication on target with an average temperature of 56.2 °C. Postoperative day 2 MRI revealed an 83 mm^3 lesion. Three-month follow-up revealed return of symptoms and absence of lesions on MRI. The following nine patients were treated at the same coordinates, but received 4–5 sonications at peak energy. Postoperative day 2 MRI revealed a 172 mm^3 lesion. At 3-month follow-up the group of nine patients showed a decrease in total UPDRS score of 60.9% and Global Symptom Relief of 56.7%. The authors reported no adverse events. In 2015, Schlesinger et al. [17] reported the results from MR-guided FUS of seven patients with tremor predominant PD. Patients underwent unilateral MR-guided FUS at standard ventralis intermedius (VIM) coordinates, 25% distance of the AC-PC anterior to the PC and 14 mm lateral to AC-PC. The thalamotomy was performed contralateral to the most disabling side. During the treatments, sonications were continued until tremors were controlled with temperature maintained below 59 °C. The authors report tremor control in all patients with a mild return of symptoms in 3 of 7 at 6 months. UPDRS at 1 week had a 50% reduction. Long-term follow-up was not reported. Several adverse events were reported, including hypogeusia, disequilibrium, and vertigo; only hypogeusia persisted past 2 months. Na et al. [23] were the first to report MRgFUS pallidotomy for PD. The patient had a 12-year history of PD and now suffered from significant

L-Dopa dyskinesias. Six months after treatment, the patient continued to have durable benefit with a 60% reduction in UPDRS Part III on medication and a 55% reduction off medication, without changes in L-Dopa equivalent daily dose. Bond et al. [15] published the first randomized controlled trial for the treatment of PD with MRgFUS. The study enrolled tremor-dominant PD patients who were randomized to two centers to receive sham vs unilateral thalamotomy. Twenty-seven patients were enrolled and six patients were assigned to the sham procedure. At 3-month follow-up mean improvement in hand tremor scores in the treatment group was 50% and 22% ($P = 0.088$) in the sham group. At 1 year, follow-up showed a tremor improvement of 40.6% ($P = 0.0154$) and mean reduction in medicated UPRDS motor scores of 3.7 (32%, $P = 0.033$). The trial showed a trend toward improvement in hand tremor and a significant reduction (improvement) of mean UPRDS scores [15].

The initial results from the use of MRgFUS for the treatment of tremor predominant PD are promising. However, it is unclear if MRgFus will fare better than DBS or established stereotactic lesioning for other types of PD. Nevertheless, the possibility of an incisionless, precise, safe treatment for medically refractory PD is compelling. Current clinical trials are underway to investigate the use of MRgFUS for traditional targets in the treatment of PD; STN, GPI, and VIM. In order to advance the use of MRgFUS in the treatment of PD, and other movement disorders, the questions that must be answered now are the same that haunted neurologists and neurosurgeons 30 years ago. What is the optimal target? What is the optimal lesion size? How do lesions compare to stimulation? Is it ever safe to perform bilateral lesions? While MRgFUS will undoubtedly have a role in the treatment of patients with PD, further trials are required to fully understand its capabilities and limitations.

References

1. Jagannathan J, Sanghvi NT, Crum LA, Yen C-P, Medel R, Dumont AS, et al. High-intensity focused ultrasound surgery of the brain: part 1--A historical perspective with modern applications. Neurosurgery. 2009;64:201–10.; discussion 210–211.
2. Christian E, Yu C, Apuzzo MLJ. Focused ultrasound: relevant history and prospects for the addition of mechanical energy to the neurosurgical armamentarium. World Neurosurg. 2014;82:354–65.
3. Krishnamoorthy VK, Sengupta PP, Gentile F, Khandheria BK. History of echocardiography and its future applications in medicine. Crit Care Med. 2007;35:S309–13.
4. Dobrakowski PP, Machowska-Majchrzak AK, Labuz-Roszak B, Majchrzak KG, Kluczewska E, Pierzchała KB. MR-guided focused ultrasound: a new generation treatment of Parkinson's disease, essential tremor and neuropathic pain. Interv Neuroradiol J Peritherapeutic Neuroradiol Surg Proced Relat Neurosci. 2014;20:275–82.
5. Fry FJ, Ades HW, Fry WJ. Production of reversible changes in the central nervous system by ultrasound. Science. 1958;127:83–4.
6. Jeanmonod D, Werner B, Morel A, Michels L, Zadicario E, Schiff G, et al. Transcranial magnetic resonance imaging–guided focused ultrasound: noninvasive central lateral thalamotomy for chronic neuropathic pain. Neurosurg Focus. 2012;32:E1.

7. Meyers R, Fry WJ, Fry FJ, Dreyer LL, Schultz DF, Noyes RF. Early experiences with ultrasonic irradiation of the pallidofugal and nigral complexes in hyperkinetic and hypertonic disorders. J Neurosurg. 1959;16:32–54.
8. Clement GT, Hynynen K. A non-invasive method for focusing ultrasound through the human skull. Phys Med Biol. 2002;47:1219–36.
9. Kuroda K. Non-invasive MR thermography using the water proton chemical shift. Int J Hyperth. 2005;21:547–60.
10. Jung HH, Kim SJ, Roh D, Chang JG, Chang WS, Kweon EJ, et al. Bilateral thermal capsulotomy with MR-guided focused ultrasound for patients with treatment-refractory obsessive-compulsive disorder: a proof-of-concept study. Mol Psychiatry. 2015;20:1205–11.
11. Elias WJ, Huss D, Voss T, Loomba J, Khaled M, Zadicario E, et al. A pilot study of focused ultrasound thalamotomy for essential tremor. N Engl J Med. 2013;369:640–8.
12. Elias WJ, Lipsman N, Ondo WG, Ghanouni P, Kim YG, Lee W, et al. A randomized trial of focused ultrasound thalamotomy for essential tremor. N Engl J Med. 2016;375:730–9.
13. Giugno A, Maugeri R, Graziano F, Gagliardo C, Franzini A, Catalano C, et al. Restoring neurological physiology: the innovative role of high-energy MR-guided focused ultrasound (HIMRgFUS). Preliminary data from a new method of lesioning surgery. Acta Neurochir Suppl. 2017;124:55–9.
14. Weintraub D, Elias WJ. The emerging role of transcranial magnetic resonance imaging-guided focused ultrasound in functional neurosurgery. Mov Disord. 2017;32(1):20–7.
15. Bond AE, Dallapiazza R, Huss D, Warren AL, Sperling S, Gwinn R, et al. A randomized, sham-controlled trial of transcranial magnetic resonance-guided focused ultrasound thalamotomy trial for the treatment of tremor-dominant, idiopathic Parkinson disease. Neurosurgery. 2016;63(Suppl 1):154.
16. Magara A, Bühler R, Moser D, Kowalski M, Pourtehrani P, Jeanmonod D. First experience with MR-guided focused ultrasound in the treatment of Parkinson's disease. J Ther Ultrasound. 2014;2:11.
17. Schlesinger I, Eran A, Sinai A, Erikh I, Nassar M, Goldsher D, et al. MRI guided focused ultrasound thalamotomy for moderate-to-severe tremor in Parkinson's disease. Park Dis. 2015;2015:219149.
18. Ghanouni P, Pauly KB, Elias WJ, Henderson J, Sheehan J, Monteith S, et al. Transcranial MRI-guided focused ultrasound: a review of the technologic and neurologic applications. AJR Am J Roentgenol. 2015;205:150–9.
19. Chang WS, Jung HH, Zadicario E, Rachmilevitch I, Tlusty T, Vitek S, et al. Factors associated with successful magnetic resonance-guided focused ultrasound treatment: efficiency of acoustic energy delivery through the skull. J Neurosurg. 2016;124:411–6.
20. Xu Z, Carlson C, Snell J, Eames M, Hananel A, Lopes MB, et al. Intracranial inertial cavitation threshold and thermal ablation lesion creation using MRI-guided 220-kHz focused ultrasound surgery: preclinical investigation. J Neurosurg. 2015;122:152–61.
21. Alkhani A, Lozano AM. Pallidotomy for parkinson disease: a review of contemporary literature. J Neurosurg. 2001;94:43–9.
22. Okun MS, Vitek JL. Lesion therapy for Parkinson's disease and other movement disorders: update and controversies. Mov Disord. 2004;19:375–89.
23. Na YC, Chang WS, Jung HH, Kweon EJ, Chang JW. Unilateral magnetic resonance–guided focused ultrasound pallidotomy for Parkinson disease. Neurology. 2015;85:549–51.

DBS Innovations in the Near Future?

12

Vignessh Kumar, Andre G. Machado,
Adolfo Ramirez-Zamora, and Julie G. Pilitsis

Introduction

Since the reported use of ventral intermediate thalamus stimulation to achieve long-term suppression of tremor by Benabid in 1991 [1] and FDA approval of deep brain stimulation (DBS) for the treatment of Parkinson's disease (PD) in 2002 [2], advances in DBS technology have opened the door to innovations in stimulation treatment. Further, as DBS technology is tested for new indications, new stimulation targets have expanded the possibilities for the future of this field. As time progresses, combinations of stimulation hardware, programming methods, novel indications, and stimulation locations can be tested to explore how DBS may be used to treat many neurological and psychiatric disorders and to determine the optimal parameters to improve patient outcomes for each of these conditions.

The primary aim of DBS innovations is to improve patient outcomes. While motor outcomes in well-selected patients are excellent, there remains a subset of motor symptoms such as gait, balance, and sleep disturbances that are not well treated [3]. Further, cognitive and psychiatric side effects may develop [4]. DBS, however, may relieve symptoms caused by medication, such as the development of

V. Kumar
Department of Neurosurgery, Albany Medical Center, Albany, NY, USA

A. G. Machado
Department of Neurosurgery, Cleveland Clinic, Neurologic Institute, Cleveland, OH, USA

Cleveland Clinic, Neurologic Institute, Center for Neurological Restoration, Cleveland, OH, USA

A. Ramirez-Zamora
Department of Neurology, University of Florida, Gainesville, FL, USA

J. G. Pilitsis (✉)
Department of Neurosurgery, Albany Medical Center, Albany, NY, USA

Department of Neuroscience and Experimental Therapeutics, Albany Medical Center, Albany, NY, USA

© Springer Nature Switzerland AG 2019
R. R. Goodman (ed.), *Surgery for Parkinson's Disease*,
https://doi.org/10.1007/978-3-319-23693-3_12

impulse control disorders (ICD) in as many as 15% of patients [5, 6]. Further, reducing medication usage improves medication-related side effects and improves quality of life [7]. Future innovations in DBS strive to reduce the burden of disease symptoms and the severity of side effects. In this chapter, we will focus on innovations in target selection, stimulator technology, and stimulator design that may become available for clinical use within the next 5 years.

Innovations in Targets

To date, DBS use in PD has primarily focused on the stimulation of the subthalamic nucleus (STN), the globus pallidus interna (GPi), and/or the ventralis intermedius (VIM) nucleus of the thalamus. While VIM DBS has been long shown to adequately control tremor in PD [8], it does not treat the other cardinal motor symptoms of PD or significantly ameliorate motor fluctuations. Thus, GPi and STN are the main two targets used, while VIM is utilized for the small percentage of tremor predominant patients at our center. It has been found that both STN and GPi DBS positively affect tremor, rigidity, bradykinesia, and freezing of gait [9–11]. While dopaminergic medications may be reduced to a greater extent after STN DBS as compared to GPi DBS, the psychiatric side effects with STN DBS may be greater [12]. Further, in patients who are exquisitely sensitive to carbidopa/levodopa, stimulation-induced dyskinesias may occur [13]. Thus, targeting depends on the individual patient [12, 14]. In our center, our default target is STN, with GPi DBS used in cases of mood/cognitive concerns, a predominant complaint of dystonia, and/or in cases of extreme sensitivity to carbidopa/levodopa.

The zona incerta (ZI), prelemniscal radiation, and subthalamic white matter fibers involved in modulating motor input, including the ansa lenticularis, thalamic fasciculus, lenticular fasciculus, and subthalamic fasciculus, have emerged as viable stimulation targets in PD. Stimulation of these targets has produced outcomes equivalent to STN and GPi stimulation in a small number of reported cases [15–17]. Further, DBS of the caudal zona incerta (cZI) was shown to better alleviate tremor in the axial musculature and limbs than stimulation of the VIM nucleus [18]. In addition to improving motor function, stimulation of the ZI was shown to enhance limbic function and alleviate depression [19].

The pedunculopontine nucleus (PPN) was reported to reduce postural instability and gait disturbances that accompany PD, in open label preliminary studies. Results of subsequent studies have been disappointing with a variety of methodological issues, including concerns with defining the appropriate patient population, appropriate outcome measures for these trials, defining the actual region stimulated, and the need of associated unilateral or bilateral STN DBS [20]. However, despite these concerns, PPN remains a potential target for treatment of PD.

Research on the stimulation of the central median-parafascicular (CM-Pf) complex, a main input and output station of the basal ganglia, shows improvement in tremor and dyskinesia [21, 22]. Although these studies recruited a small number of patients, they demonstrated that CM-Pf DBS did not cause prominent cognitive or psychiatric adverse effects. Future large-scale studies will provide a better insight into the clinical effectiveness of this new target.

Recently, stimulation of the substantia nigra reticulata (SNr) has been explored as a potential target for the alleviation of refractory postural instability and impaired locomotion in PD. In animal models, high frequency stimulation (HFS) of the SNr improves forelimb akinesia, postulated to be through the attenuation of SNr neuronal activity, increase in VM thalamic neuron activity, and decrease of SNr beta oscillations, suggesting that the SNr may be a plausible DBS target for treatment of motor symptoms in PD [23]. Bilateral stimulation of the SNr pars reticulate improved axial Parkinsonian motor symptoms (specifically, gait and balance disorders) with an increase in braking capacity but had no effect on distal Parkinsonian motor symptoms [24]. It is believed that overactive GABAergic inhibitory inputs cause excessive inhibition of the midbrain locomotion region in PD, leading to subsequent gait failure. SNr-HFS may reduce this excess inhibition by downregulating SNr neuronal activity. In a double-blind, randomized, cross-over, controlled clinical trial, 12 patients with PD received either simultaneous stimulation of the STN and SNr (programmed with interleaved pulses) or standard STN-DBS [25]. The global, broad primary endpoint revealed no significant improvement of axial motor functioning with combined STN and SNr stimulation, but investigators observed improved freezing of gait with combined stimulation. Further studies evaluating concomitant STN and SNr stimulation for intractable freezing of gait are needed.

While the stimulation of specific neural targets can lead to the improvement of certain characteristics of PD, simultaneous stimulation of multiple targets may produce better effects than single-target stimulation. Stefani et al. have shown that simultaneous stimulation of the PPN and STN allows for improved alleviation of the motor, gait, and postural symptoms of PD as compared to stimulation of either the PPN or STN alone [20]. Furthermore, studies have demonstrated that synchronous DBS stimulation of multiple areas allows for cross-talk, the formation of a circuit between these regions. Neural circuitry developed as a result of cross-talk has been shown to be frequency-dependent [26].

The relative advantages, adverse effects, and interactions with medications observed with stimulation of emerging PD DBS targets will dictate the future implementation of these targets. As research continues to unveil benefits and drawbacks of targets that make certain stimulation areas best suited for specific patient preferences, the feasibility of routinely employing these stimulation targets can be further explored.

Innovations in Technology

Innovation and enhancement of DBS technology can allow for adverse effects of stimulation to be minimized. In particular, advances in electrode design and implantable device hardware will allow for increased stimulation resolution or "directional stimulation," preventing "stimulation spillage" into adjacent areas and decreasing the incidence of side effects from unintended stimulation.

Regardless, accurate placement of the stimulation electrode is essential to DBS efficacy [27]. However, preoperative stereotactic imaging for electrode guidance often is not sufficient for the accurate placement of electrodes [28]. For this reason, most surgeons supplement stereotactic imaging with microelectrode recording [27] and other methods of target localization. Magnetic resonance imaging (MRI)-guided electrode placement was shown to improve motor symptoms [29] without inducing some of the side effects seen with MER-guided electrode placement [29–32]. Use of MRI-guided DBS has drawn attention to the use of different sequences, which may allow for better target visualization, such as Fast Gray Matter Acquisition T1 Inversion Recovery (FGATIR) [28]. In addition, diffusion tensor imaging (DTI), traditionally used for the localization of white matter, has emerged as a way of predicting the efficacy of stimulation by determining the proximity of the DBS electrode to efferent white matter tracts [33]. Effective stimulation of white matter tracts has been recognized to have growing importance in targeting [34]. Further, it has allowed an improved understanding of connections between regions [35, 36].

Innovations in Electrode Design

In order to achieve optimal stimulation, DBS electrodes must be designed specific to two important factors: (1) the disease and (2) the characteristics of the target tissue. The electric field pattern (EFP) and the volume of tissue activated (VTA) are variables that can be manipulated to best address these two factors. In order to identify the ideal EFP and VTA for certain targets of stimulation, computer models can be generated to test a wide array of electrode shapes and dimensions [37].

The concept of computer-assisted shape-optimization has recently been applied to develop an electrode ideally suited for VIM DBS. A cylindrical contact with length 2.54 mm and diameter of 0.75 mm produces a VTA that activates 54% of the VIM nucleus, as opposed to the standard electrode VTA that activates 26% of the VIM nucleus [37]. Future applications of this technology involve modeling other stimulation targets, such as the STN and GPi, as well as electrode design optimization to achieve maximal activation of the target area. The generation of computer models prior to implantation of the DBS system may allow for more patient-centric, personalized treatment.

Regulation of EFP and VTA can be achieved through the specification of electrode directionality, which is shaping the pattern of current flow around the lead. While traditional leads have EFPs that emanate in a ring shape from the electrode, it is possible to engineer electrodes with a skewed EFP, designed such that stimulation is not symmetrical with respect to the electrode's central axis [38]. This technique will allow for tissue activation to be more specific, maximizing the beneficial effects of accurate target stimulation and minimizing the adverse effects of undesired stimulation of nearby tissue (see Fig. 12.1). Traditional ring-EFP electrodes and altered EFP electrodes are differentiated by electrode

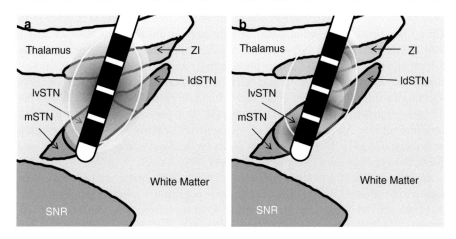

Fig. 12.1 The use of current steering (**b**) allows for controlled stimulation of the STN, as opposed to the unspecific stimulation of neighboring tissue in traditional stimulation (**a**). ZI, zona incerta; ldSTN, latero-dorsal subthalmic nucleus; SNR, recticular substantia nigra; lvSTN, latero-ventral subthalmic nucleus; mSTN, medial subthalmic nucleus

resolution. Greater electrode resolution can be achieved through advances in nanotechnology and microfabrication [39, 40] to produce electrodes with more specific areas of activation. The implementation of DBS arrays (the arrangement of DBS electrodes in various patterns) allows the combined EFP to assume a noncircular shape [38]. Directionality of individual electrodes may be used to further shape the field.

Further directionality may be achieved with each electrode being independently powered [41]. It has been hypothesized that this advance may allow for better adaptation to impedance changes as well. Whether constant current devices or spatial steering properties offer further advantages has yet to be validated [38, 42].

Closed-Loop Systems

The future of DBS holds great promise in technology that can adapt to the patient. Traditional stimulation parameters are programmed to an unchanging intensity, unresponsive to fluctuating activity in the brain. Stimulation-induced side effects, such as alterations in motor and cognitive function, can be reduced through the adjustment of stimulation parameters in response to feedback from neural targets [43]. Methods of generating feedback for responsive stimulators include the detection of neurotransmitter concentrations, the measurement of target firing (local field potentials), and the detection of limb movement through external devices. Response to electrical signals is likely the first step [44].

A goal of a closed-loop system would be to deliver stimulation at the appropriate time, to avoid supra- or sub-therapeutic stimulation, by responding to patterns or rates of activity, ideally in the same area where the DBS electrode is in place [45]. Thus, appropriate stimulation could be delivered during different tasks or at rest [46]. For instance, while GPi-DBS can facilitate transition from the akinetic state toward movement initiation, it may unnecessarily stimulate non-motor circuits that control key cognitive functions and behavior. Responsive technology could allow for "on demand" stimulation. These technologies may also be beneficial due to the progressive nature of PD, so the device would ideally be able to adapt to changing neuronal activity. An added benefit of "on demand" systems would be preservation of battery life [47]. Devices to treat epilepsy in this fashion are available and Tourette's syndrome is a likely next target [48, 49].

In PD, local field potentials (LFPs), a measure of electrical activity, have been shown to be altered [50, 51]. Specifically, there is greater oscillatory neuronal firing and beta activity [50]. The use of closed-loop monitoring to compare LFPs in patients with PD to normal LFP data may allow for stimulation parameters to adapt to changes in the activity of neuronal populations. Figure 12.2 shows sample STN LFP data for a patient between the eyes closed (2A) and eyes open (2B) states, demonstrating the feasibility of LFP recording.

The Wireless Instantaneous Neurotransmitter Concentration System (WINCS) is a tool used for real-time monitoring of dopamine concentrations [52]. The integration of WINCS with DBS hardware will allow for the adaptation of stimulation intensity in response to fluctuations in local dopamine levels. Implanting the WINCS monitoring device at the site of projections of target neurons might ensure dopamine concentrations are maintained at proper physiological levels, eliminating the adverse effects of over- and under-stimulation.

Another option is the use of external sensors that measure muscle activity, either through surface-electromyography (sEMG) or through sensors that track and analyze limb movement [53]. sEMG quantifies limb movement though the detection of muscle contractions. This has potential use in movement disorders. Before external

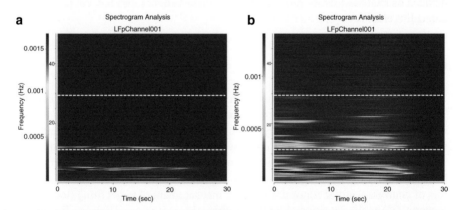

Fig. 12.2 Spectograms of a single patient's subthalmic nucleus LFP complete recordings. The lower segment highlights the alpha range (8 Hz–12 Hz); the middle segment the low beta range (13–20 Hz); and the upper segment the high beta range (21–29 Hz). (**a**) represents eyes closed, (**b**) represents eyes open

sensors can be implemented, they must be designed such that they are small enough to wear and can wirelessly transmit information to the implantable pulse generator (IPG). Accelerometers small enough to wear on the wrist are widely used as pedometers. The commonplace nature of wearable accelerometers suggests that these devices have potential applications in monitoring tremor activity, as has been attempted in patients with epilepsy [54]. Wireless transmission of signals from the sEMG/accelerometer to the pulse generator, while feasible, must use a radio-frequency receiver small enough to fit within the implanted device. Although external sensors have not yet been implemented, their noninvasive properties make them a promising solution for closed-loop systems.

Optogenetics

Despite the well-documented benefits of DBS, the mechanism of DBS action remains unclear [55]. Recent developments in the field of optogenetics have led to the elucidation of DBS mechanisms [56, 57]. Optogenetics involves the use of genetic modification and viral transduction to induce the expression of light-sensitive proteins in specific neuronal populations, allowing for these neurons to be activated in response to light [58]. Thus, the illumination of a certain brain area will only activate neurons that express light-sensitive proteins, leading to more specific activation than can be achieved with stimulation from electric current [57].

Optogenetics has catalyzed the identification of pathways that are essential to alleviation of PD symptoms by STN-DBS [56, 58]. Multiple studies in transgenic mouse models have demonstrated that the reduction of PD symptoms is not caused by activation of STN cell bodies, but instead the activation of STN afferents [56, 58], such as tracts connecting the M1 motor region to the STN [56]. These results indicate that the therapeutic benefits derived from DBS are likely caused by DBS-induced changes in the M1-STN pathway [57]. Whether optogenetics will be used clinically remains dependent on progress with cell-specific targeting and viral transduction [57].

Summary
- The impetus behind advances in DBS technology is to increase DBS efficacy and minimize adverse effects associated with DBS.
- Advances in imaging are useful in predicting efficacy of stimulation and understanding connections between relevant regions.
- Advances in electrode design allow for optimization of the electric field pattern (EFP) and volume of tissue activated (VTA), improving intended stimulation while decreasing spillage.
- Closed-loop stimulation and responsive technology can reduce periods of supra- and sub-therapeutic stimulation without manual adjustment of stimulation parameters.

Innovations in Programming

DBS programming parameters consist of cathode selection, anode selection, and amplitude, pulse width (PW), and frequency settings. The quantity and quality of stimulation is dictated by the combination in which these variables are applied and are individualized for the patient. Although recommended programming algorithms have been published [59], differences in patients' individual regional anatomy, lead location, clinical phenotype, and propensity to experience side effects mandate individualized programming assessments. While previous research has primarily focused on altering amplitude to produce maximal effects from DBS, similar manipulations to PW and frequency are now being investigated [60]. Effects on battery life and development of adverse effects should be considered [60].

Optimal stimulation requires the use of pulse widths that are specific to the properties of target tissue, as different stimulation targets have varying levels of excitability. This property of neural tissue is measured by the chronaxie, defined as the minimum amount of time a target must be stimulated for it to be activated. Thus, a tissue with a larger chronaxie is less excitable. For example, DBS chronaxie was shown to be 75 μs for stimulation of the GPi and 65 μs for stimulation of the thalamus [61, 62]. The larger chronaxie of the GPi indicates that a greater pulse width must be used to achieve optimal target excitation. On the other hand, increases in frequency up to 130 Hz have shown to be beneficial to patient outcomes in VIM DBS [59].

The utility of conventional programming techniques might be limited by the occurrence of common side effects, including dysarthria, dyskinesia, and other motor symptoms, as previously demonstrated [63]. Interleaved stimulation (ILS) is a novel approach of optimizing the stimulation field to provide maximal symptom alleviation, while minimizing the adverse effects of stimulation. ILS allows for two programs to be interleaved in an alternating fashion on the same lead, with each program driving its own combination of active electrodes, pulse width, and amplitude [64]. Interleaved stimulation can provide adequate control of PD symptoms while mitigating the negative effects of stimulation. Recent studies have demonstrated the benefits of interleaved stimulation in the management of refractory dysarthria, Parkinsonism, and dyskinesias while avoiding side effects with a step-by-step algorithm approach [65]. Battery life is a concern with interleaved stimulation, as specific settings might increase battery drain. Long-term efficacy and battery life studies are needed to establish the effectiveness of ILS.

Another potential option is burst stimulation, where a brief high frequency train of pulses is integrated into traditional programming parameters [66] (see Fig. 12.3). Although burst stimulation has not been incorporated into routine DBS, preliminary evidence from its use in spinal cord stimulation (SCS) has demonstrated its effectiveness [66, 67].

Gene Therapy

The applications of gene therapy in the treatment of PD have rapidly been explored since 2010 with mixed results, with novel regulation of molecular targets in animal models showing promise in restoring dopaminergic transmission

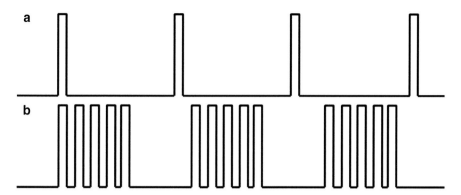

Fig. 12.3 Waveforms of (**a**) traditional stimulation and (**b**) burst stimulation. Burst stimulation, while maintaining the sample amplitude and pulse width, features electrical impulses delivered at periods of high frequency

[68]. Transition of gene therapy techniques to human patients is relatively recent, with the first human clinical trials conducted having been conducted in 2014 [69] and newer studies suggesting logistic advantages of combining the invasive nature of gene therapy administration with simultaneous DBS lead implantation [70].

Local restoration of dopamine production in the striatum is one avenue of approach in the use of gene therapy in alleviation of PD. A 15-patient trial was conducted to assess the efficacy of administering a lentiviral vector designed to reestablish striatal dopamine production [69]. The viral vector was administered into the putamen bilaterally, and PD outcomes and adverse effects were monitored. While UPDRS III motor scores off medication were shown to significantly improve at 6 months and 12 months compared to baseline, on-medication dyskinesias (11 patients) and on-off phenomena (9 patients) were reported [69]. Long-term patient follow-up showed evidence of clinical benefit and tolerability up to 4 years following treatment. While the results of this first-in-human clinical trial carry a tone of initial optimism, the authors caution that the increase in UPDRS III motor scores seen in this investigation are within the placebo range reported in other clinical trials [69, 71, 72].

The role of neurotrophic factors in normal neural physiology and the treatment of PD continue to be explored. Various neurotrophic factors, including glial derived neurotrophic factor (GDNF), neurturin, cerebral dopamine neurotrophic factor, and mesencephalic astrocyte-derived neurotrophic factor, have shown both protective and restorative potential in preserving and enhancing dopamine transmission [73]. In a rodent model, upregulated expression of GDNF was shown to have both neuroprotective and neurorestorative effects on dopaminergic circuitry in a 6-hydroxydopamine model (6-OHDA) of PD [68].

Although in its infancy, the application of gene therapy in the treatment of PD is a developing therapeutic option with its efficacy soon to be evaluated in forthcoming clinical trials. The combination of gene therapy with DBS and medical management affords a greater number of therapeutic options for the management of PD in the future.

Conclusion

The future of deep brain stimulation and its applications in Parkinson's disease will stem from combined innovations in electrode technology, pulse generator technology, stimulation parameters, and targeting. These improvements may improve the efficacy of DBS for all patients with Parkinson's disease as well as allow for customization of technologies and techniques toward specific symptoms profiles. Additionally, this experience will further the use of DBS in other diseases and for other symptoms. It is an exciting time to be in neuromodulation as we explore the potential of these technologies.

References

1. Benabid AL, Pollak P, Gervason C, Hoffmann D, Gao DM, Hommel M, Perret JE, de Rougemont J. Long-term suppression of tremor by chronic stimulation of the ventral intermediate thalamic nucleus. Lancet. 1991;337:403–6.
2. Gardner J. A history of deep brain stimulation: technological innovation and the role of clinical assessment tools. Soc Stud Sci. 2013;43(5):707–28.
3. McColl CD, Reardon KA, Shiff M, Kempster PA. Motor response to levodopa and the evolution of motor fluctuations in the first decade of treatment of Parkinson's disease. Mov Disord. 2002;17:1227–34.
4. Gopinathan G, Teravainen H, Dambrosia JM, Ward CD, Sanes JN, Stuart WK, Evarts EV, Calne DB. Lisuride in parkinsonism. Neurology. 1981;31:371–6.
5. Lhommee E, Klinger H, Thobois S, Schmitt E, Ardouin C, Bichon A, Kistner A, Fraix V, Xie J, Aya Kombo M, Chabardes S, Seigneuret E, Benabid AL, Mertens P, Polo G, Carnicella S, Quesada JL, Bosson JL, Broussolle E, Pollak P, Krack P. Subthalamic stimulation in Parkinson's disease: restoring the balance of motivated behaviours. Brain. 2012;135:1463–77.
6. Weintraub D, Siderowf AD, Potenza MN, Goveas J, Morales KH, Duda JE, Moberg PJ, Stern MB. Association of dopamine agonist use with impulse control disorders in Parkinson disease. Arch Neurol. 2006;63:969–73.
7. Martinez-Martin P, Valldeoriola F, Tolosa E, Pilleri M, Molinuevo JL, Rumia J, Ferrer E. Bilateral subthalamic nucleus stimulation and quality of life in advanced Parkinson's disease. Mov Disord. 2002;17:372–7.
8. Benabid AL, Pollak P, Louveau A, Henry S, de Rougemont J. Combined (thalamotomy and stimulation) stereotactic surgery of the VIM thalamic nucleus for bilateral Parkinson disease. Appl Neurophysiol. 1987;50:344–6.
9. Anderson VC, Burchiel KJ, Hogarth P, Favre J, Hammerstad JP. Pallidal vs subthalamic nucleus deep brain stimulation in Parkinson disease. Arch Neurol. 2005;62:554–60.
10. Krause M, Fogel W, Heck A, Hacke W, Bonsanto M, Trenkwalder C, Tronnier V. Deep brain stimulation for the treatment of Parkinson's disease: subthalamic nucleus versus globus pallidus internus. J Neurol Neurosurg Psychiatry. 2001;70:464–70.
11. Schupbach WM, Chastan N, Welter ML, Houeto JL, Mesnage V, Bonnet AM, Czernecki V, Maltete D, Hartmann A, Mallet L, Pidoux B, Dormont D, Navarro S, Cornu P, Mallet A, Agid Y. Stimulation of the subthalamic nucleus in Parkinson's disease: a 5 year follow up. J Neurol Neurosurg Psychiatry. 2005;76:1640–4.
12. Odekerken VJ, van Laar T, Staal MJ, Mosch A, Hoffmann CF, Nijssen PC, Beute GN, van Vugt JP, Lenders MW, Contarino MF, Mink MS, Bour LJ, van den Munckhof P, Schmand BA, de Haan RJ, Schuurman PR, de Bie RM. Subthalamic nucleus versus globus pallidus bilateral

deep brain stimulation for advanced Parkinson's disease (NSTAPS study): a randomised controlled trial. Lancet Neurol. 2013;12:37–44.

13. Lyons MK. Deep brain stimulation: current and future clinical applications. Mayo Clin Proc. 2011;86:662–72.

14. Weaver FM, Follett KA, Stern M, Luo P, Harris CL, Hur K, Marks WJ Jr, Rothlind J, Sagher O, Moy C, Pahwa R, Burchiel K, Hogarth P, Lai EC, Duda JE, Holloway K, Samii A, Horn S, Bronstein JM, Stoner G, Starr PA, Simpson R, Baltuch G, De Salles A, Huang GD, Reda DJ, Group CSPS. Randomized trial of deep brain stimulation for Parkinson disease: thirty-six-month outcomes. Neurology. 2012;79:55–65.

15. Desiraju T, Purpura DP. Synaptic convergence of cerebellar and lenticular projections to thalamus. Brain Res. 1969;15:544–7.

16. Jimenez F, Velasco F, Velasco M, Brito F, Morel C, Marquez I, Perez ML. Subthalamic prelemniscal radiation stimulation for the treatment of Parkinson's disease: electrophysiological characterization of the area. Arch Med Res. 2000;31:270–81.

17. Velasco F, Jimenez F, Perez ML, Carrillo-Ruiz JD, Velasco AL, Ceballos J, Velasco M. Electrical stimulation of the prelemniscal radiation in the treatment of Parkinson's disease: an old target revised with new techniques. Neurosurgery. 2001;49:293–306. discussion 306-298.

18. Plaha P, Ben-Shlomo Y, Patel NK, Gill SS. Stimulation of the caudal zona incerta is superior to stimulation of the subthalamic nucleus in improving contralateral parkinsonism. Brain. 2006;129:1732–47.

19. Burrows AM, Ravin PD, Novak P, Peters ML, Dessureau B, Swearer J, Pilitsis JG. Limbic and motor function comparison of deep brain stimulation of the zona incerta and subthalamic nucleus. Neurosurgery. 2012;70:125–30. discussion 130-121.

20. Stefani A, Lozano AM, Peppe A, Stanzione P, Galati S, Tropepi D, Pierantozzi M, Brusa L, Scarnati E, Mazzone P. Bilateral deep brain stimulation of the pedunculopontine and subthalamic nuclei in severe Parkinson's disease. Brain. 2007;130:1596–607.

21. Jouve L, Salin P, Melon C, Kerkerian-Le Goff L. Deep brain stimulation of the center median-parafascicular complex of the thalamus has efficient anti-parkinsonian action associated with widespread cellular responses in the basal ganglia network in a rat model of Parkinson's disease. J Neurosci. 2010;30:9919–28.

22. Stefani A, Peppe A, Pierantozzi M, Galati S, Moschella V, Stanzione P, Mazzone P. Multi-target strategy for Parkinsonian patients: the role of deep brain stimulation in the centromedian-parafascicularis complex. Brain Res Bull. 2009;78(2–3):113–8.

23. Sutton AC, Yu W, Calos ME, Smith AB, Ramirez-Zamora A, Molho ES, Pilitsis JG, Brotchie JM, Shin DS. Deep brain stimulation of the substantia nigra pars reticulata improves forelimb akinesia in the hemiparkinsonian rat. J Neurophysiol. 2013;109:363–74.

24. Chastan N, Westby GW, Yelnik J, Bardinet E, Do MC, Agid Y, Welter ML. Effects of nigral stimulation on locomotion and postural stability in patients with Parkinson's disease. Brain. 2009;132:172–84.

25. Weiss D, Walach M, Meisner C, Fritz M, Scholten M, Breit S, Plewnia C, Bender B, Gharabaghi A, Wachter T, Kruger R. Nigral stimulation for resistant axial motor impairment in Parkinson's disease? A randomized controlled trial. Brain. 2013;136:2098–108.

26. Liu X, Ford-Dunn HL, Hayward GN, Nandi D, Miall RC, Aziz TZ, Stein JF. The oscillatory activity in the parkinsonian subthalamic nucleus investigated using the macro-electrodes for deep brain stimulation. Clin Neurophysiol. 2002;113:1667–72.

27. Amirnovin R, Williams ZM, Cosgrove GR, Eskandar EN. Experience with microelectrode guided subthalamic nucleus deep brain stimulation. Neurosurgery. 2006;58:ONS96–102. discussion ONS196-102.

28. Sudhyadhom A, Haq IU, Foote KD, Okun MS, Bova FJ. A high resolution and high contrast MRI for differentiation of subcortical structures for DBS targeting: the fast gray matter acquisition T1 inversion recovery (FGATIR). NeuroImage. 2009;47(Suppl 2):T44–52.

29. Foltynie T, Zrinzo L, Martinez-Torres I, Tripoliti E, Petersen E, Holl E, Aviles-Olmos I, Jahanshahi M, Hariz M, Limousin P. MRI-guided STN DBS in Parkinson's disease without microelectrode recording: efficacy and safety. J Neurol Neurosurg Psychiatry. 2011;82:358–63.
30. Ben-Haim S, Asaad WF, Gale JT, Eskandar EN. Risk factors for hemorrhage during microelectrode-guided deep brain stimulation and the introduction of an improved microelectrode design. Neurosurgery. 2009;64:754–62. discussion 762-753.
31. Binder DK, Rau GM, Starr PA. Risk factors for hemorrhage during microelectrode-guided deep brain stimulator implantation for movement disorders. Neurosurgery. 2005;56:722–32. discussion 722-732.
32. Hariz MI, Fodstad H. Do microelectrode techniques increase accuracy or decrease risks in pallidotomy and deep brain stimulation? A critical review of the literature. Stereotact Funct Neurosurg. 1999;72:157–69.
33. Gross RE, McDougal ME. Technological advances in the surgical treatment of movement disorders. Curr Neurol Neurosci Rep. 2013;13:371.
34. Deniau JM, Degos B, Bosch C, Maurice N. Deep brain stimulation mechanisms: beyond the concept of local functional inhibition. Eur J Neurosci. 2010;32:1080–91.
35. Lambert C, Zrinzo L, Nagy Z, Lutti A, Hariz M, Foltynie T, Draganski B, Ashburner J, Frackowiak R. Confirmation of functional zones within the human subthalamic nucleus: patterns of connectivity and sub-parcellation using diffusion weighted imaging. NeuroImage. 2012;60:83–94.
36. Traynor CR, Barker GJ, Crum WR, Williams SC, Richardson MP. Segmentation of the thalamus in MRI based on T1 and T2. NeuroImage. 2011;56:939–50.
37. Butson CR, McIntyre CC. Role of electrode design on the volume of tissue activated during deep brain stimulation. J Neural Eng. 2006;3:1–8.
38. Martens HCF, Toader E, Decre MMJ, Anderson DJ, Vetter R, Kipke DR, Baker KB, Johnson MD, Vitek JL. Spatial steering of deep brain stimulation volumes using a novel lead design. Clin Neurophysiol. 2011;122:558–66.
39. Cheung KC. Implantable microscale neural interfaces. Biomed Microdevices. 2007;9: 923–38.
40. Rodger DC, Fong AJ, Wen L, Ameri H, Ahuja AK, Gutierrez C, Lavrov I, Hui Z, Menon PR, Meng E, Burdick JW, Roy RR, Edgerton VR, Weiland JD, Humayun MS, Tai YC. Flexible parylene-based multielectrode array technology for high-density neural stimulation and recording. Sens Actuators B Chem. 2008;132:449–60.
41. Butson CR, McIntyre CC. Current steering to control the volume of tissue activated during deep brain stimulation. Brain Stimul. 2008;1:7–15.
42. Okun MS, Gallo BV, Mandybur G, Jagid J, Foote KD, Revilla FJ, Alterman R, Jankovic J, Simpson R, Junn F, Verhagen L, Arle JE, Ford B, Goodman RR, Stewart RM, Horn S, Baltuch GH, Kopell BH, Marshall F, Peichel D, Pahwa R, Lyons KE, Troster AI, Vitek JL, Tagliati M, Group SDS. Subthalamic deep brain stimulation with a constant-current device in Parkinson's disease: an open-label randomised controlled trial. Lancet Neurol. 2012;11:140–9.
43. Lee KH, Blaha CD, Garris PA, Mohseni P, Horne AE, Bennet KE, Agnesi F, Bledsoe JM, Lester DB, Kimble C, Min HK, Kim YB, Cho ZH. Evolution of deep brain stimulation: human electrometer and smart devices supporting the next generation of therapy. Neuromodulation. 2009;12:85–103.
44. Van Gompel JJ, Chang SY, Goerss SJ, Kim IY, Kimble C, Bennet KE, Lee KH. Development of intraoperative electrochemical detection: wireless instantaneous neurochemical concentration sensor for deep brain stimulation feedback. Neurosurg Focus. 2010;29:E6.
45. Bergman H, Wichmann T, Karmon B, DeLong MR. The primate subthalamic nucleus. II Neuronal activity in the MPTP model of parkinsonism. J Neurophysiol. 1994;72:507–20.
46. DeLong MR. Activity of pallidal neurons during movement. J Neurophysiol. 1971;34:414–27.
47. Herron J, Chizeck H. Prototype closed-loop deep brain stimulation systems inspired by Norbert Wiener. 2014 IEEE Conference on Norbert Wiener in the 21st Century (21CW). 2014. p. 1–6.

48. Morrell MJ, Group RNSSiES. Responsive cortical stimulation for the treatment of medically intractable partial epilepsy. Neurology. 2011;77:1295–304.
49. Okun MS, Foote KD, Wu SS, Ward HE, Bowers D, Rodriguez RL, Malaty IA, Goodman WK, Gilbert DM, Walker HC, Mink JW, Merritt S, Morishita T, Sanchez JC. A trial of scheduled deep brain stimulation for Tourette syndrome: moving away from continuous deep brain stimulation paradigms. JAMA Neurol. 2013;70:85–94.
50. Kuhn AA, Trottenberg T, Kivi A, Kupsch A, Schneider GH, Brown P. The relationship between local field potential and neuronal discharge in the subthalamic nucleus of patients with Parkinson's disease. Exp Neurol. 2005;194:212–20.
51. Toledo JB, Lopez-Azcarate J, Garcia-Garcia D, Guridi J, Valencia M, Artieda J, Obeso J, Alegre M, Rodriguez-Oroz M. High beta activity in the subthalamic nucleus and freezing of gait in Parkinson's disease. Neurobiol Dis. 2014;64:60–5.
52. Agnesi F, Tye SJ, Bledsoe JM, Griessenauer CJ, Kimble CJ, Sieck GC, Bennet KE, Garris PA, Blaha CD, Lee KH. Wireless instantaneous neurotransmitter concentration system-based amperometric detection of dopamine, adenosine, and glutamate for intraoperative neurochemical monitoring. J Neurosurg. 2009;111:701–11.
53. Shukla P, Basu I, Graupe D, Tuninetti D, Slavin KV. A neural network-based design of an on-off adaptive control for deep brain stimulation in movement disorders. Conf Proc IEEE Eng Med Biol Soc. 2012;2012:4140–3.
54. Lockman J, Fisher RS, Olson DM. Detection of seizure-like movements using a wrist accelerometer. Epilepsy Behav. 2011;20:638–41.
55. Lee KH, Chang SY, Jang DP, Kim I, Goerss S, Gompel J, Min P, Arora K, Marsh M, Hwang SC, Kimble CJ, Garris P, Blaha C, Bennet KE. Emerging techniques for elucidating mechanism of action of deep brain stimulation. Conf Proc IEEE Eng Med Biol Soc. 2011;2011:677–80.
56. Gradinaru V, Mogri M, Thompson KR, Henderson JM, Deisseroth K. Optical deconstruction of parkinsonian neural circuitry. Science. 2009;324:354–9.
57. LaLumiere RT. A new technique for controlling the brain: optogenetics and its potential for use in research and the clinic. Brain Stimul. 2011;4:1–6.
58. Lobo MK, Nestler EJ, Covington HE 3rd. Potential utility of optogenetics in the study of depression. Biol Psychiatry. 2012;71:1068–74.
59. Volkmann J, Moro E, Pahwa R. Basic algorithms for the programming of deep brain stimulation in Parkinson's disease. Mov Disord. 2006;21(Suppl 14):S284–9.
60. Moro E, Esselink RJ, Xie J, Hommel M, Benabid AL, Pollak P. The impact on Parkinson's disease of electrical parameter settings in STN stimulation. Neurology. 2002;59:706–13.
61. Holsheimer J, Demeulemeester H, Nuttin B, de Sutter P. Identification of the target neuronal elements in electrical deep brain stimulation. Eur J Neurosci. 2000;12:4573–7.
62. Holsheimer J, Dijkstra EA, Demeulemeester H, Nuttin B. Chronaxie calculated from current-duration and voltage-duration data. J Neurosci Methods. 2000;97:45–50.
63. Umemura A, Oka Y, Yamamoto K, Okita K, Matsukawa N, Yamada K. Complications of subthalamic nucleus stimulation in Parkinson's disease. Neurol Med Chir (Tokyo). 2011;51:749–55.
64. Barbe MT, Dembek TA, Becker J, Raethjen J, Hartinger M, Meister IG, Runge M, Maarouf M, Fink GR, Timmermann L. Individualized current-shaping reduces DBS-induced dysarthria in patients with essential tremor. Neurology. 2014;82:614–9.
65. Ramirez-Zamora A, Kahn M, Campbell J, DeLaCruz P, Pilitsis JG. Interleaved programming of subthalamic deep brain stimulation to avoid adverse effects and preserve motor benefit in Parkinson's disease. J Neurol. 2015;262:578–84.
66. De Ridder D, Vanneste S, Plazier M, van der Loo E, Menovsky T. Burst spinal cord stimulation: toward paresthesia-free pain suppression. Neurosurgery. 2010;66:986–90.
67. De Ridder D, Plazier M, Kamerling N, Menovsky T, Vanneste S. Burst spinal cord stimulation for limb and back pain. World Neurosurg. 2013;80:642–649 e1.
68. Tereshchenko J, Maddalena A, Bahr M, Kugler S. Pharmacologically controlled, discontinuous GDNF gene therapy restores motor function in a rat model of Parkinson's disease. Neurobiol Dis. 2014;65:35–42.

69. Palfi S, Gurruchaga JM, Ralph GS, Lepetit H, Lavisse S, Buttery PC, Watts C, Miskin J, Kelleher M, Deeley S, Iwamuro H, Lefaucheur JP, Thiriez C, Fenelon G, Lucas C, Brugieres P, Gabriel I, Abhay K, Drouot X, Tani N, Kas A, Ghaleh B, Le Corvoisier P, Dolphin P, Breen DP, Mason S, Guzman NV, Mazarakis ND, Radcliffe PA, Harrop R, Kingsman SM, Rascol O, Naylor S, Barker RA, Hantraye P, Remy P, Cesaro P, Mitrophanous KA. Long-term safety and tolerability of ProSavin, a lentiviral vector-based gene therapy for Parkinson's disease: a dose escalation, open-label, phase 1/2 trial. Lancet. 2014;383:1138–46.
70. Rowland NC, Starr PA, Larson PS, Ostrem JL, Marks WJ Jr, Lim DA. Combining cell transplants or gene therapy with deep brain stimulation for Parkinson's disease. Mov Disord. 2015;30:190–5.
71. Christine CW, Starr PA, Larson PS, Eberling JL, Jagust WJ, Hawkins RA, VanBrocklin HF, Wright JF, Bankiewicz KS, Aminoff MJ. Safety and tolerability of putaminal AADC gene therapy for Parkinson disease. Neurology. 2009;73:1662–9.
72. Marks WJ Jr, Ostrem JL, Verhagen L, Starr PA, Larson PS, Bakay RA, Taylor R, Cahn-Weiner DA, Stoessl AJ, Olanow CW, Bartus RT. Safety and tolerability of intraputaminal delivery of CERE-120 (adeno-associated virus serotype 2-neurturin) to patients with idiopathic Parkinson's disease: an open-label, phase I trial. Lancet Neurol. 2008;7:400–8.
73. Domanskyi A, Saarma M, Airavaara M. Prospects of neurotrophic factors for Parkinson's disease: comparison of protein and gene therapy. Hum Gene Ther. 2015;26:550–9.

Index

© Springer Nature Switzerland AG 2019
R. R. Goodman (ed.), *Surgery for Parkinson's Disease*,
https://doi.org/10.1007/978-3-319-23693-3